A GUIDE TO CLINICAL DRUG RESEARCH

A GUIDE TO CLINICAL DRUG RESEARCH
SECOND EDITION

edited by

ADAM COHEN
Professor of Clinical Pharmacology,
University of Leiden,
Leiden, The Netherlands
and
Director of the Centre for Human Drug Research,
Leiden University Hospital,
Leiden, The Netherlands

and

JOHN POSNER
Independent Consultant
in Pharmaceutical
Medicine

Springer

Library of Congress Cataloging-in-Publication Data

A guide to clinical drug research / edited by Adam Cohen and John Posner.—2nd ed.
p. : cm
Includes bibliographical references and index.
ISBN 0-7923-6171-7
1. Drugs—Research. 2 Drugs—Testing. I. Cohen, Adam. II. Ponser, John.
[DNLM: 1. Clinical Trials—methods. 2. Research Design. QV 771 G946 2000]
RM301.27.G85 2000
615'.19—dc21

99-089541

ISBN 0-7923-6172-5

Cohen & Posner: A Guide to Clinical Drug Research, Second Edition

First Indian Reprint 2009

ISBN 978-81-8489-310-6

This edition is manufactured in India for sale only in India, Pakistan, Bangladesh, Nepal and Sri Lanka and any other country as authorized by the publisher.

This edition is published by Springer (India) Private Limited, (a part of Springer Science+Business Media), Registered Office: 3rd Floor, Gandharva Mahavidyalaya, 212, Deen Dayal Upadhyaya Marg, New Delhi – 110 002, India.

Printed in India by Rakmo Press (P) Ltd., New Delhi.

Contents

Foreword to the first edition

Clinical drug research forms the experimental basis for efficacy and safety assessment of new therapeutic agents in man. In other words, it allows us to obtain relevant information on how to effectively and safely use a drug in an individual patient. Clinical research is a of key importance for developing and validating new concepts in clinical pharmacology and therapeutics, using already existing and new biologically active agents. Increasingly, it is also conducted to compare different treatment regimens in order to reveal that one is superior to another.

In recent years clinical drug research has advanced strongly with the availability of new pharmacokinetic, pharmacodynamic and clinical methods and sophisticated ethical and quality assurance standards, automated and on line data management. This has made such research much more efficient and informative. The quality of the information to be obtained depends on a clear definition of the question to be answered or hypothesis to be tested, a scientifically sound concept has to be translated into an appropriate study design, protocol and data evaluation. Dissemination of the information obtained using the appropriate channels should also be considered an important objective of any study.

This book is a 'Guide to Clinical Drug Research' in the literal sense of the word. It provides the reader with relevant information about every aspect of drug research in man, from the initial research idea to the ultimate publication and with every step in between.

The Editors, who started their career working together at the clinical pharmacology department of the Wellcome Research Laboratories in Beckenham, are very experienced in clinical drug research and very knowledgeable about what is needed to perform such research to up-to-date standards. They have managed to successfully involve a number of colleagues working in clinical pharmacology or other departments in the pharmaceutical industry. In addition, experts from other fields have written about important topics.

This book is not only of importance for scientists and other persons engaged in clinical drug research. Much of the principles and technical aspects discussed are relevant for any type of clinical research. The use of this knowledge in any clinical research project will undoubtedly lead to improved quality and relevance.

Douwe D.Breimer, Ph.D.
Professor of Pharmacology,
Director of Research of the Leiden/Amsterdam
Center for Drug Research, Leiden University

Editor's notes to the second edition

Since the publication of the first edition guidelines for the conduct of pre-clinical and clinical research have been agreed by the USA, Europe and Japan under the auspices of the International Conference of Harmonisation (ICH). These developments have been reflected in revision of certain chapters. Other chapters are virtually unchanged. Additions to the book include a brief new chapter on Clinical Study reports and a glossary of commonly used terms.
The internet has become an important means of communication for clinical investigators as well as drug research in the past four years but we have resisted the temptation to include references to 'interesting' wedsites recognising that they would become rapidly outdated. Despite the fast rate of change in pharmaceutical research and development, the principles of clinical drug research are generally unchanged. We therefore trust that the book will remain a useful primer for those in academia setting out on the path of becoming an investigator in clinical research and will help to fill the gaps for those with more experience in the field.

John Posner and Adam Cohen
Editors

Glossary of commonly used terms

Adverse event The ICH defines an adverse event as: *"Any untoward medical occurrence in a patient or clinical investigation subject administered a pharmaceutical product and which does not necessarily have to have a causal relationship with this treatment"* (see ICH Guideline: Clinical safety data management: definitions and standards for expedited reporting). For non-marketed drugs, or new indications of marketed drugs, an adverse event is referred to as an adverse drug reaction when there is a reasonable possibility that it was caused by the medicinal product, i.e. a causal relationship cannot be ruled out.

Biomarker A measure that is an indicator of a normal physiologic process, or a pathologic state or the response of an organism to an intervention that can be used in drug research. When a biomarker can replace a clinical endpoint it is called a surrogate endpoint.

Clinical Drug Development. Phases This classification assumes a sequential approach to drug development. However, the clinical pharmacology programme will overlap the later phases with a number of studies that are required for registration (e.g. interaction studies, or studies in special populations – elderly, renally or hepatically-impaired), and are performed at the same time as the Phase II/III studies.

Phase I Clinical Pharmacology
Studies in healthy volunteers (sometimes patients) to determine the safety and tolerability of the drug, other dynamic effects and the pharmacokinetic profile (absorption, distribution, metabolism and excretion – ADME). Evidence of efficacy may be gained if patients, disease models or biomarkers are used.

Phase II Clinical Investigation
Early studies in patients with the target disease, to determine efficacy, safety and tolerability in carefully controlled dose-ranging studies

Phase III Formal clinical trials
Large-scale placebo controlled and active comparator studies in patients to confirm efficacy, and provide further information on the safety and tolerability of the drug.

Phase IV Post-marketing surveillance to expand safety and efficacy data in a large population, including further formal therapeutic trials and comparisons with other active comparators

Clinical endpoint A measure of how a patient feels, functions or survives.

Clinical Investigator's Brochure An extensive summary of all that is known about a research compound with regard to pre-clinical and clinical data.

Ethics Committee An independent group of professionals often complemented by a non-scientific member of the public responsible for approval of study protocols before a study is actually carried out. Subject safety and scientific integrity of the protocol are the main concerns.

Good Clinical Practice A standard to ensure protection of research subjects and data integrity in clinical studies of new drugs.

International Conference on Harmonisation The International Conference on Harmonisation (ICH) has produced guidelines on Good Clinical Practice (GCP) encompassing the requirements of the European Union (EU), Japan and the United States (US) as well as those of the World Health Organisation (WHO), Australia, New Zealand and the Nordic Countries (ICH Topic E6, Guidelines on Good Clinical Practice).

Investigator A suitably trained scientist (often medically qualified) involved in the execution of a clinical drug study. The person with ultimate responsibility for this is called principal or responsible investigator

Pharmacodynamics The scientific discipline involved in the study of drug action on molecular or cellular targets or on the whole organism.

Pharmaco-kinetics	The study of the time course of the concentration of a substance and its metabolites in body fluids like blood and urine.
Pre-clinical Drug Development	The studies done in cells, tissues and whole animals as well as the chemical and pharmaceutical investigations to obtain adequate assurance that a new drug may safely given to man in clinical studies.
Quality Assurance	The procedures and control systems in place during a clinical trial to ensure integrity of the data and protection of subjects.
Quality Control	The checks performed to ensure that the quality control system is adhered to.
Serious Adverse Event (SAE)	An adverse event that leads to death, permanent disability or (prolongation of) hospital admission. These events are of obvious importance to authorities and fellow researchers working on the same drug and have to be reported to the local and international authorities with the greatest possible urgency. The details of the reporting are given in the study protocol.
Sponsor	An organisation (often a pharmaceutical company) funding a trial of a new drug or other intervention for registration purposes .
Standard Operating Procedure (SOP)	A detailed description of a certain activity or organising principle in a clinical trial. Such procedures must be adhered to when performing a trial under the Good Clinical Practice standards.
Study Protocol	The document describing the rationale, the patient population, the drugs to be used and the full time schedule of a clinical study as well as the endpoints to be evaluated. The study protocol with the investigator's brochure is given to the Ethics Committee for independent evaluation.
Surrogate endpoint	A biomarker that has been extensively studied to be sufficiently confident that it can replace a clinical endpoint for registration purposes.

List of contributors

Nigel S. Baber,
MB, BSc, FRCP, FFPM
Clinical Pharmacologist
Medicines Control Agency
London, UK
Chapter 3

Peter van Brummelen, MD, PhD
Research Director
Yamanouchi Europe BV
Leiderdorp, the Netherlands
Chapter 12

Karin Overbeek, Msc,
Chief librarian
Yamanouchi Europe BV
Leiderdorp, the Netherlands
Chapter 12

Adam F. Cohen, MD, PhD
Professor of Clinical Pharmacology
CHDR Leiden
Zernikedreef 10
2333 CL Leiden, The Netherlands
Editor

Nicola La Grue
Head of Medical Writing Dept
Bios (Consultancy & Contract Research Ltd)
Bagshot, Surrey, UK
Chapter 13

William P. Howlett,
DTM&H, FRCP(I), PhD
Consultant Physician
Kilimanjaro Christian Medical Centre.
Moshi, Tanzania
Chapter 14

Les Huson, PhD
Medical statistician
Roche Global development
Welwyn, UK
Chapter 7

Gregor B. E. Jemec, MD
Assistant Professor of Dermatology
Bispeberg Hospital
University of Copenhagen
DK_2400 Copenhagen, Denmark
Chapter 9

Ria Kroon, BSc
Quality Assurance Manager
CHDR
Zernikedreef 10
2333 CL Leiden, The Netherlands
Chapter 11

Alfred H.J. van Meurs
Consultant Paediatrician
Kilimanjaro Christian Medical Centre
Moshi, Tanzania
current address:
Juliana Children's Hospital
The Hague, The Netherlands
Chapter 14

Fiona Peachy, PhD
International Project Manager
Glaxo Wellcome PLC
Beckenham, Kent , UK
Chapter 8

John Posner, BSc, PhD, FRCP, FFPM
Independent Consultant in Pharmaceutical Medicine, UK
Editor

Patricia Sohl, MD
Nyhavn 45_IFAL
DK_1051 Kopenhagen, Denmark
Chapter 9

Jean Soul-Lawton
Clinical Research Scientist
Glaxo Wellcome PLC
Greenford, Middx, UK
Chapter 11

Steve Warrington, MA, MD, FRCP, FFPM
Medical Director
Hammersmith Medicines Research Ltd.
London, UK
Chapter 10

1

Clinical research: From idea to publication

A.F.Cohen and J. Posner

Introduction

This book is about the practical aspects of performing clinical drug research starting from the conception of an idea through to publication of a completed piece of research in a peer reviewed scientific journal. In the last two or three decades it has become progressively more difficult to perform good clinical research. There are a number of reasons for this:

- The volume of scientific literature published is now so vast that it is easy to miss important pieces of research which might impact on the project of interest to you.
- As the cost of health care rises, concern about the cost-effectiveness of therapeutic agents and strategies has increased. It is no longer good enough to demonstrate that a new medication is relatively safe and effective; rather it is necessary to provide evidence that it is superior to another treatment or even that there is an advantage over not treating the patient at all. This means that clinical trials with drugs have become larger and more costly and consequently harder to perform.
- Concerns about protection of subjects in clinical trials and fears of scientific fraud have led to a situation in which the development and licensing of new medicines has become highly regulated. Good Clinical Practice (GCP) and Good Laboratory Practice (GLP) have certainly contributed to the quality of medical research but place an enormous burden on the clinical researcher both in terms of resources and sheer complexity. Great care must be taken to ensure that all the activities necessary to perform successful clinical research do not compromise patient care. There are times when ethical issues may arise in reconciling these two.

The first medicines were given for diseases of which the pathophysiology was fairly well understood and for which the indicators of therapeutic efficacy were clear. Thus, in 1948 a trial of streptomycin for the treatment of tuberculosis (generally considered to be the first controlled clinical trial) only required 109 patients to achieve its objectives. Nowadays, many infections can be cured by drugs or prevented with vaccines, hypertension, thyroid disorders and even epilepsy can usually be controlled quite well. The endpoints are now much more difficult to achieve, such as the reduction of secondary myocardial infarction or mortality by long term intervention with a particular treatment strategy. The current therapeutic challenges are among others, diseases like cancer, rheumatoid arthritis, Alzheimer's dementia, septic shock and multiple sclerosis. The pathophysiology of these conditions is often poorly understood and complex therapeutic strategies are usually required. The scale of work involved in determining the efficacy of these strategies is much greater. The ISIS IV study, which investigated three different drugs alone and in combination for the treatment of myocardial infarction required almost 60,000 patients! The complexity of these studies demands a multidisciplinary approach. This has changed the clinical scientist from somebody who could work almost single-handed to a manager of a large group of people and considerable financial resources.

Anyone wanting to start a new research project is obviously best advised to do this in an established environment with experience in all operational aspects of performing clinical drug research. However this is not always possible and individual researchers are faced with the unenviable task of discovering for themselves, expending a great deal of effort on reinventing the wheel. Just as a travel guide allows you to visit a town more effectively than by rediscovering all important sites by yourself, this guide should ensure a more rapid entry into the field of clinical research. The emphasis will be on drug research but the principles and most of the detail should be applicable to all types of clinical research.

The generation of ideas

It is not difficult to have good ideas for clinical research. Whilst still students or during the course of carrying out their clinical duties most doctors are curious about why they do what they do to patients or why a particular disease behaves as it does. Likewise, scientists working in a medical field will be inquisitive by nature and training. This curiosity, the wanting to know 'how' or 'why' is the basis of all ideas for research.

Limiting and focussing ideas

When you have an idea, write it down as soon as possible. Some people have fleeting ideas at unpredictable moments, while driving home from work or in the middle of the night. It pays to write them down in a rough format so that they won't be forgotten. At this stage you should be not too restrictive in what you write down; limit what you write to two or three sentences at most. This tends to set limits and focuses the idea. If the idea still looks exciting when you look at it the next day, continue with the next stage.

Generating a specific hypothesis that can be tested

If the hypothesis is not defined early in the life of the idea it may be extremely painful. For example if you submit a research proposal that is extremely broad, it is unlikely to attract funding as it may be unclear what the project will yield. Additionally it is generally difficult to attract collaborators for such a project as most people will find it too vague and open ended. Cutting down the project when you have taken the trouble to develop a full research proposal can represent a large waste of effort and money.

A workable hypothesis should be phrased like a question. There are obviously no hard rules for this but generally a good hypothesis is a question that has a relatively simple answer. To get a feel for what constitutes a well phrased hypothesis, take a recent issue of a medical journal like the New England Journal of Medicine or The Lancet and extract the hypotheses from some of the papers.

Processing ideas

Not all ideas are good and, like the raw ingredients required to make a good meal, they can be acquired fairly easily but no one will appreciate them without a lot of further processing. Although there are rare individuals who are capable of processing their own ideas, most of us need to be challenged by others and obtain their views and contributions to them so that they can be sifted and refined. This is needed because the amount of energy required to actually perform a drug study is much greater than that required to generate the original idea. It is likely that you will have many more ideas than can ever be tested and the processing of ideas will allow you to select projects with the greatest chance of success. Unlike the food processor which can be bought from a shop, the 'ideas processor' needs to be built from a group of individuals involved in research. Once established, the most successful clinical researcher will value such a group above all else as it will allow him to use his limited manpower and resources on the most promising projects.

So, the 'ideas processor' is a group of people that discusses new ideas. There are no set rules about the composition of the group or how it operates. It is very dependent on the type of research that is undertaken, the organisation in which you work, existing traditions and the personality of the people involved. It is essential that the prime aim of the group is kept in sight at all times, namely to apply a selection process to any ideas or proposals so that no further time or effort are spent on unpromising ideas. Of course opinions may differ about the value of a particular idea and the fact that someone holds a minority view doesn't mean that they are wrong. The history of medicine and science teach us that some of the most outstanding breakthroughs have been made by individuals who have had heretical ideas and been in a minority of one. Nevertheless, if everyone in the group is committed to the genuine evaluation of all ideas however preposterous they may sound at first and whoever thought them up, the process will work effectively. A consensus can often be obtained if there is an ethos of mutual trust and respect. The group should not operate in a very formal manner receiving research proposals that are described in great detail. Processing of unpolished ideas should take place at a very early stage in an informal atmosphere.

Perhaps you are worried by all this talk about ideas. Maybe you don't seem to have had many ideas and even fewer good ones. Possibly you have never considered yourself an original and creative thinker. This doesn't mean you cannot be a clinical researcher and participate in the ideas processing group. An effective group may make you realise that you are really a creative individual and that your ideas just needed a little coaxing.

Alternatively, it may help you to appreciate that your real talents lie in constructive criticism and refining of other people's raw ideas. Or perhaps you excel in the actual performance of studies, while the ideas generators may not be very good in practicalities and attention to detail. The ideas processing group should enable each member of the team to fulfil themselves in the role at which they are best.

Has someone else had the same idea?

At this stage of processing it may look as if your idea was good. Unfortunately that means that someone else has probably had the same idea and results may have already been published. There is no excuse for missing a relevant publication and for this it is essential that you have access to a well equipped library which takes most of the journals published in medicine and the biological sciences. As well as following up references by pulling books and journals off the shelves you should make use of computerised literature searches like MEDLINE or CD-ROM or any of the search facilities provided on the internet. If you do not have ready access to these facilities you may be able to operate by mail or through a colleague in another country.

If you have been working in a field for a long time you may know exactly what everyone else is doing through going to meetings and from other researchers in your group. If you want to enter a new area it is useful to speak to established researchers in that field and ask for their opinion. You may be worried that these people will copy your idea and competition can be fierce in some areas but most established researchers are busy and cannot easily change their plans. In addition they may be quite pleased to collaborate.

Has the question really been answered before?

Often someone did have the idea first but they did not achieve their objectives or answer the question adequately. To evaluate this, you will need to learn to read scientific papers carefully and develop your analytical and critical faculties. At the end of this chapter a checklist is given which may be used in this evaluation process; with experience you may decide to develop your own checklist. Assuming that no one else had your idea before or if they did the question was not adequately resolved, you continue with the next stage.

What do you want your research to accomplish?

You may not be at all sure what is a realistic expectation but it is sensible to have a goal in sight. Could it result in a major change in clinical practice or is it to characterise some aspect of a drug which will help it obtain a product license or improve the way we use a marketed product? Is it intended to answer a more basic science question such as how a drug or endogenous substance works or to gain a better understanding about the pathophysiology of a disease process? Will it help us to gain a better understanding of the epidemiology of a disease?

Which journal might publish your results?

Once you are clear about the general goal, you can start to think about journals that may publish your results. If you hope that the results of your research will have an impact on clinical practice, you will need to have very convincing data. The study must be of sufficient size and of robust design and the endpoints must be applicable to patient populations. It was known for more than 30 years that aspirin affected platelet function before a very large study was performed which resulted in the drug being used routinely after myocardial infarction! If you plan for success, you should aim for publication in a first line general medical journal or one specialising in the relevant field. Research of a more basic scientific nature should generally be directed at specialist clinical or basic biological science journals.

Pharmaceutical companies and some scientific institutions sponsor much of the research on potential new medicines and many that are already on the market. The wishes of the sponsor will need to be taken into account when considering when and where to publish and the conditions attached to publication will generally form part of the contract between you and the sponsor. Results of clinical trials are usually published in general medical and specialist clinical journals although there are now journals dedicated specifically to clinical trials. Studies of pharmacodynamics and pharmacokinetics are generally published in clinical pharmacology journals. Much of this research also forms part of the clinical section of dossiers submitted as applications for product licenses to regulatory authorities.

The first study

As the result of processing your ideas and critically evaluating the published literature, you will have outlined the clinical research project. This may consist of a series of studies in humans supported by in vitro experiments and in vivo studies in animals. It probably won't be possible to define some of the later studies precisely as they will be dependent on results of earlier work. Sooner or later the moment of truth arrives; it is time to write a summary or concept sheet of the first study you want to perform. It is useful to use a standard format; it should not be longer than two A4 sheets of paper otherwise nobody will read it. A suggested structure is as follows:

- **Background and rationale**
  This describes briefly why it is necessary to perform the study. If you have followed the initial processing steps it should not be difficult to write this section as it summarises all your previous considerations about the idea. Ethical aspects may be considered here for the first time.
- **Objectives**
  The specific objectives of the study are extremely important. There should be a limited number, certainly no more than three and they should be stated as clearly and briefly as possible.
- **Study population**
  This section will define the entry and exclusion criteria in the protocol. You may indicate age ranges, sex, diagnosis, etc. and you may have an initial idea about the number of subjects.
- **Main endpoints**
  Here you state what you suppose your main study endpoints are going to be. These should be the key measurements and comparisons to be made which will support or refute your hypothesis. It could be mortality at a predefined timepoint or a sophisticated endocrinological measurement or plasma concentrations of a drug.
- **Outline of procedures and schedule**
  At this stage, it probably won't be possible to define precise times of blood samples or tests but it is sensible to put down some idea of how many days or weeks the study will take, what procedures will be performed and how often.
- **Statistical aspects**
  In the first instance this may be left open, but it should be there to remind you of the necessity to address this

point as soon as possible.

This rough summary is used for further discussions with your ideas processing group. After these discussions you probably will want to write the summary again and it should now contain a lot more detail. Such a cyclical approach to the development of a protocol may seem inefficient at first but makes a lot of sense for clinical research proposals that require the input from many people. You will find that some of your colleagues or superiors will only be stimulated to think seriously about the proposal when they see a sketchy outline!

As the details of the execution of the study are discussed a useful device is to write the paper in advance. This may sound like scientific fraud but of course you are not actually putting in real data; it simply forces you to think in terms of results and what they might mean. It may even be possible to draw some graphs and make tables containing both expected and unexpected results. With these you can do 'What if?' exercises. Such simulations may lead to changes in the design of the study.

Resources

At this point your idea has been processed into a study and you are almost ready to write the protocol. Before proceeding, there are some important resource issues that need to be addressed. The detailed planning and budgeting are described in Chapter 5 but you should now consider the following points:

- **Staff**

  At the early stages of a project it is easy to imagine that you can do everything yourself. Generally this is not the case and you are likely to need nurses and physicians, administrative staff, computer programmers and statisticians. They may need training and time needs to be allowed for this.
- **Equipment**

  Equipment is always readily available until it is needed for the study! At that point it will be required for routine clinical use or for an emergency or will have been sent away for repairs. It may be necessary to acquire special diagnostic equipment, computers or laboratory

CHECKLIST FOR ASSESSING CLINICAL TRIALS
(from Weintraub, 1990 with permission)

TITLE:

GENERAL CHARACTERISTICS

Objective: Major ____________________

Subsidiary (1) ____________________

(2) ____________________

Phase: ☐ I ☐ II ☐ III☐ IV ☐ Other
Type: ☐ Experiment ☐ Survey ☐ Prospective ☐ Retrospective
Design: ☐ Within patient (crossover, Latin square, or randomised blocks)
☐ Between patient (one way, parallel groups)

SPECIFIC CHARACTERISTICS	Discussed?	Evaluation/Comment	Problems
Population			
Type (patients/healthy)			
Rationale for size (n)			
Expected difference			
How recruited?			
Inclusion criteria			
Exclusion criteria			
Comparability of groups			
Demographic			
Prognostic criteria			
Stage of disease			
Response to therapy			
Associated disease			
Similarity to usual patients			
Treatments Compared			
Dose rationale and details			
Amount/time			
Amount/kg;other			
Fixed or flexible			
One dose level			
Dosage form, route			
Duration of therapy			
Ancillary therapy			
Biopharmaceutics			
Source (lot number)			
Bioavailability			
Test medication			
Standard medication			
Appearance			

SPECIFIC CHARACTERSTICS	Discussed?	Evaluation/Comment	Problems
Eperimental Design			
Controls			
Active or inactive			
Concurrent or historical			
Test medication added to current treatment?			
Factorial design			
Assignment of treatments			
Randomised?(balanced?)			
Stratification?			
Other			
Run in or washout period			
Timing (schedule of visits, laboratory tests)			
Data collection			
Measurements used to assess goal			
Observers (Who? Variable?)			
Method of collection			
Adverse effects			
Subjective (Volunteered, elicited)			
Objective			
Bias control			
"Blind" observers			
"Blind" subjects			
Evaluator blind but observer non-blind			
Statistician's analysis			
Results			
Primary outcome measure			
Secondary outcome measures			
Adverse reactions			
Drop-outs or drop-ins			
Reasons			
Effect on results			
Compliance			
Investigators			
Subgroup analysis			
Predictors of response			
Data Analysis			
Comparability of treatment groups			
Missing data			
Compliance taken into account			
Statistical tests			
Differences			
No difference due to limited power?			

OVERALL ASSESSMENT

Any "fatal" errors that invalidate results? ☐ Yes ☐ No

Conclusions justified? ☐ Yes ☐ No

GENERAL COMMENTS:

apparatus for the project. Delivery of specialist equipment can take a long time.

- **Space**
  You may need office or laboratory space in addition to the clinical facilities where the study will be conducted (see Chapter 2). After the study has started no one will believe you need it, so think about your needs early. If space has to be rented, this has implications for your budget.
- **Patients/Subjects**
  The availability of subjects for your clinical study remains an important point of attention throughout the project but it is better dealt with from the start.
- **Time**
  You need a realistic time schedule for the study. Most projects take longer than the most pessimistic predictions. You may have moved on to another job before it is finished; the continuity of the project needs to be thought about at the start.

Having done all this work you now have a well prepared project. There are many further steps which should help to make the project a success. They are described in more detail in the rest of this book.

2

Facilities and Equipment

J. Posner and A.F.Cohen

Introduction

The facilities in which clinical research is conducted obviously vary enormously with circumstances. High quality research which has far reaching consequences can be performed in some of the poorest countries in the world using the most basic facilities. Conversely, research of inferior quality is sometimes performed in teaching hospitals and purpose-built contract research organisations in the West. Nevertheless, it is common sense that failure to be adequately equipped to meet the requirements of conducting a specific study in humans will have a negative impact on the quality of data obtained and is likely to compromise the safety of the subjects. The Association of the British Pharmaceutical Industry (ABPI) has therefore issued guidelines on minimum standards for facilities for the conduct of studies in non-patient volunteers and, in our view, these standards are applicable to most clinical research that is conducted on inpatients as well. While these guidelines are not legally binding there are certainly medico-legal implications for clinicians conducting research in conditions which do not meet the requirements and everyone involved in such activities should be familiar with them. It should also be recognised that, if the results of the study are submitted to a regulatory authority such as the Food and Drug Administration (FDA) in the USA, the data are quite likely to be unacceptable simply because of inadequate compliance with Good Clinical Practice (see Chapter 11). It therefore behoves every clinical researcher to be sure that the facilities in which he conducts research are adequate. What follows is not intended to substitute for any existing guidelines but summarises and briefly discusses the standards that should be met.

Facilities

Ideally, the building in which clinical research is conducted on healthy volunteers or patients should be designed for this purpose. It is extremely difficult to carry out complex procedures and intensive blood sampling on a general hospital ward. If such a facility is not available the accommodation should be modified so that subjects are comfortable and staff can conduct the research in a safe and proficient manner. Consideration should be given to the fact that study subjects are entitled to privacy and that confidentiality is a requirement of Good Clinical Practice; therefore the general public should not have access to the Unit.

If not situated in a hospital, the facility should have easy access for an ambulance and be within a few minutes drive of a hospital capable of handling emergencies. Corridors and doorways should be sufficiently wide to allow passage of a bed or stretcher. It should be appreciated that even if a clinical study is being conducted in a medical school or hospital building, access to emergency staff and facilities is not guaranteed. A little back room at the top of a flight of stairs is not an appropriate location for this sort of activity.

The ward area should be separate from those where subjects and staff eat or prepare meals so that there is no chance of contaminating food with biological specimens. Its layout must be such that staff can monitor the well being of all subjects easily. Single rooms with subjects hidden behind closed doors or curtains are not compatible with close observation at all times. There should be adequate space for medical and nursing staff to administer the study out of ear shot but at close proximity to the subjects. Even if it is not intended for a study to be residential, the facilities should provide for an overnight stay for subjects and staff in the event of a subject feeling unwell or not being fit for discharge at the end of the study day.

Biological samples should be handled and stored in a separate, designated room which meets the requirements of Health and Safety standards and Good Clinical Practice. Toilet facilities should be adequate taking into account that subjects may be required to provide accurately timed urine or faecal specimens and collections. There should be a secure cupboard for storage of drugs at room temperature and a secure refrigerator designated exclusively for storage of drugs which must be stored under these conditions. Appropriate arrangements must be made for the additional security required for storage and accountability of controlled drugs. There should be adequate arrangements with the local pharmacy for formulation, storage and dispensing of drugs. If it is absolutely necessary to prepare formulations in the Unit, this should be done in a clean area or room designated for the purpose.

Emergency equipment

Apart from apparatus that may be required for carrying out specific tests and investigations, the facility should be equipped to monitor the wellbeing of subjects and to cope with emergencies. This should include the following:

- An emergency electricity supply for lighting and appliances
- An alarm call system within the unit and clear arrangements and procedures for summoning help by telephone, bleep etc from outside the unit
- Tilting beds and adequate space around each bed to cope with emergencies
- Equipment to monitor and record blood pressure and electrocardiograms
- An emergency medical oxygen supply with adequate equipment for its delivery
- A defibrillator, suction apparatus, laryngoscope, ambubag or other masks etc for assisted ventilation
- Intravenous fluids and drugs to cope with cardiac arrest and arrhythmias, acute pulmonary oedema, hypoglycaemia, opiate-induced narcosis, acute allergic responses, anaphylaxis and acute bronchospasm; other specific antidotes to drugs being studied may also be appropriate

Procedures should be in place for regular checking of all the above equipment and replacement of drugs that have gone beyond their expiry dates. Most importantly, staff must undergo regular training in use of the equipment. All staff including non-medical personnel who work in the facility should have a course in basic life support with regular refreshers ideally every six months. Physicians should also receive advanced life support training though it is important that all personnel should know their limitations and be able to summon help quickly rather than undertake procedures that are beyond their level of competence. Arrangements should be in place to transfer an unwell subject to hospital as quickly as possible.

Comprehensive records should be kept of all equipment checks and training.

As all personnel responsible for delivery of healthcare will know, proficient handling of emergencies has at least as much to do with being prepared for the simple things that are so liable to go wrong. It is only with regular rehearsals that one can discover that the physician on call doesn't always have his bleep switched on, that a particular nurse is slow to summon help or has forgotten how to switch on the defibrillator, that there are no spare batteries for the laryngoscope or that a connector for mask and tubing is missing.

Support services

The safe and efficient conduct of clinical research is always dependent on a number of support services. These include:

- An ethics committee
- Insurance and legal advice
- Clinical pathology and other laboratories
- Catering and domestic staff

A properly constituted Ethics Committee is essential for compliance with the Declaration of Helsinki (see Chapter 9) and consequently with GCP. The Ethics Committee should not only review the study protocol but will generally have inspected the facilities where the work will be carried out.

Medically qualified personnel must be insured and the academic institution or company should be indemnified against damages caused to subjects and staff participating in a study. If arrangements are not in place for this, the advice of insurance and legal experts on such matters is well worth seeking. It is also advisable that, in addition to the Ethics Committee, a legal expert review the content and specific wording of the consent form (see Chapter 9).

Almost all clinical studies involve the services of a clinical pathology laboratory for haematology and biochemistry. In the past, hospital services were often taken for granted both with respect to the fact that tests performed to support the research were often not paid for and the quality controls were presumed to be adequate. Now, most laboratories will, quite reasonably charge for tests that would not have been performed as part of the routine clinical care of the patient. This of course opens them up to competition and private external laboratories may sometimes be less expensive. What is more important, however, is whether the standards of the laboratory comply with Good Laboratory Practice and that the quality, reporting and interpretation of data are of the highest order. It is essential that the laboratory is staffed and equipped to support research activities in terms of quantity of samples to be handled, adequacy of controls and normal ranges of the population being studied.

Archives It is a requirement of Good Clinical Practice that, when a study is complete, all documentation relating to that trial should be archived and kept for a very long time, dependent upon the time of marketing authorisation for a compound in different countries. If the study is being conducted on behalf of a drug company, the company will usually insist on you passing over all the files and they will archive them. If not sponsored in this way, you may be tempted to consider this unnecessary but there are sound reasons for this practice to be recommended for all clinical studies. This may be of particular importance in view of impending legislation for clinical trials in many European countries. You may wish to access some of the data at a later date, however unlikely this may seem at the time and there are medicolegal implications of conducting experiments on humans. The documentation should include a copy of the protocol with any amendments, final report/publication, all correspondence relating to the study, the case report forms including results of blood tests, electrocardiograms and other tests, laboratory note books and computer disks (see Chapter 5). Particularly for large or prolonged studies, it is advisable to catalogue and archive the documents while the study is still in progress.

The problem of space for housing the archive always arises. Ideally, the archive should be held in a fireproof cabinet in a room which is secure. If you are very industrious and complete several studies in a year or a study involves many hundreds of patients, the storage space required may be much larger than can be accommodated in a single cabinet. A suitable room or building for the archive will need to be found and fitted out appropriately. One way of saving space and safeguarding your data against fire and theft is to use microfilm.

Approximately 6,000 double-sided pages will fit on a single reel of microfilm of 2 by 5 by 5 cm which can be computer indexed. The reading equipment can be used to print pages. It is acceptable to destroy the originals, but you must have detailed procedures in place to safeguard the completeness of the microfilm record. Digital imaging and storage of documents is also now possible, but this too requires careful procedures to ensure completeness and the ability to retrieve the documents in the future.

Further reading

- Association of the British Pharmaceutical Industry: Guidelines on standards for the facilities in which studies on non-patient volunteers are conducted.
- European Guidelines on Resuscitation and Advanced Life Support.
- Guidelines on Good Clinical Practice.

3

What does the investigator need to know about the drug?- the Clinical Investigator's Brochure.

Nigel Baber

Introduction

This chapter describes what you, as an investigator, should know before conducting a clinical study. Before you embark on any study, you should be assured that the sponsoring pharmaceutical company has provided a complete description of the investigational product in the form of an up to date Clinical Investigator's Brochure. Usually the product under investigation is a drug, as this chapter assumes, but it should be remembered that information about a novel device for drug administration should undergo equal scrutiny.

The study may be a first administration of a new chemical entity (NCE), in which case only pre-clinical information can be supplied. Alternatively, it may be a post-registration support study with clinical data on several thousand patients being available. Whatever the phase of drug development you must be able to interpret all the information on the drug that has been supplied, before the protocol is submitted to the Ethics Review Committee (ERC) or Institutional Review Board (IRB), and before asking subjects to participate in the study.

The chapter concentrates on what you need to know prior to a Phase I study, with emphasis on the toxicological requirements before human exposure, and early human pharmacokinetic and pharmacodynamic data. The extra information that is usually available prior to later phase trials will be described in less detail.

As an investigator you should be aware of your responsibilities, and those of the sponsoring company, to act in accordance with GCP. Those pertinent to the information on study drugs are summarised below:

- Sponsor's responsibilities

The sponsor should ensure that sufficient safety and efficacy data from non-clinical studies and/or clinical trials are available to support human exposure by the route, at the dosages, for the duration, and in the trial population to be studied. Information on any comparator agents used must also be provided.

The sponsor should provide the investigator with the protocol and an up-to-date Clinical Investigators Brochure (CIB), and should provide sufficient time for the investigator to review this information. The sponsor must also inform the investigator of any relevant new information arising during the trial.

- Investigator's responsibilities

The investigator should be thoroughly familiar with the appropriate use of the investigational product (and any comparators), as described in the protocol, in the current CIB, in the product information, and in other information sources provided by the sponsor. It is the investigator's responsibility to provide the appropriate EC(s)/IRB(s) with an up-to-date CIB.

Sources of Information

The main source of information on the drug is likely to be the CIB. However, there are a number of other useful sources that may be available.

Details of the clinical development plan for the drug may be confidential, but it is useful to find out where the current study lies in the overall strategy for the drug's evaluation. The Introduction or Rationale sections of the protocol may summarise this information.

Relevant publications should be obtained, as these may support the rationale for the drug's development and/or the specific study. They may also give valuable clues to possible safety, dynamic or kinetic characteristics of the drug to be studied, particularly if they describe experiences with drugs of the same or similar class.

Face-to face meetings with clinical representatives of the sponsor are particularly helpful, and if the drug is in the early stages of development it is useful if a pre-clinical representative can attend these meetings. In the case of multi-centre studies it is usual to have an investigator's meeting. Meetings with the sponsor should be used as an opportunity to raise any outstanding concerns about the drug, as well as dealing with procedural issues relating to study conduct.

It is important to ascertain whether other investigators have turned down the study, and if so, why. It is also very important to know of any previous EC or IRB refusals, the reasons given, and the actions taken. Likewise, have there been any regulatory problems?

The Clinical Investigator's Brochure

In accordance with GCP, the Investigator should be provided with a CIB containing the essential information on the drug. For studies with licensed drugs, or late phase studies, a data sheet or technical monograph may be supplied instead of a CIB. Safety information about all indications and presentations of the study drug should be presented, even if the CIB supports a specific indication or presentation.

The CIB should be concise, objective and non-promotional in order to allow the reader to make an unbiased risk-benefit assessment of the drug and its suitability for study in human subjects.

The CIB should provide a summary description of:

- the formulation and physical properties of the drug (stability, solubility, pH etc.)
- the pharmacological and toxicological effects in animals and human subjects
- the pharmacokinetics of the drug in animals and human subjects
- the safety and effectiveness in human subjects known to date
- any possible risks and adverse effects
- any precautions or special monitoring required with the use of the drug, including overdose management

This information should be adequate to justify the nature, scale and duration of the trial you are being asked to perform.

CIBs should be reviewed and revised if necessary at least annually. When reviewing a CIB you should note the date of issue, and request a summary of any data that has been generated since this date. It is your responsibility to provide an up to date CIB to the EC/IRB.

A detailed list of contents of a CIB is presented in Box

3.1, which could be used as a checklist when you review data supplied by the sponsoring drug company.

Box 3.1 Contents of a Clinical Investigator's Brochure

General description of the drug
Physical properties (form and appearance, solubility, formula)
Chemical properties
Pharmaceutical properties (strength of dosage forms, composition, storage requirements and stability)

Pre-clinical section

- **Pharmacology**
  Specific pharmacology
  General pharmacology
  Safety pharmacology
  Metabolism and pharmacokinetics in animals
- **Toxicology**
  Single and repeated dose studies
  Toxicokinetics
  Carcinogenicity (if appropriate)
  Reproductive studies
  Genotoxicity

Clinical section

- **Clinical Pharmacology (Phase I)**
  Safety
  Tolerability
  Pharmacokinetics
  Metabolism (including radiolabelled studies)
  Pharmacodynamics (biological effect, including surrogate marker effect)
  Interactions (kinetic and dynamic)
  Special groups (e.g. elderly, hepatic or renal impairment)
- **Clinical Research (Phase II & III)**
  Clinical safety
  Clinical efficacy (dose-response in placebo-controlled studies, active comparator studies)

References
Publications and reports

Summary of data and guidance to investigators

General description of the drug

Details of the relevant physical, chemical and pharmaceutical properties of the drug and its formulation should be provided in the CIB. You should pay particular attention to the following information:

- Presentation of the drug (and active or placebo comparator)
  For double-blind studies it is important that the study drug and comparator preparations are as identical as possible in all respects – appearance, taste and texture.

- Storage conditions, stability and shelf-life
  Some materials must be stored under strict conditions, at a certain temperature or humidity, or away from direct sunlight for example. Products also have a shelf-life since they may degrade over time and require reanalysing for potency and purity. On receiving the clinical supplies you should check the expiry date against the expected completion date of your study. It is very inconvenient to discover that your drug supplies are unusable in the middle of a clinical trial.

- Handling instructions (including reconstitution instructions if necessary)
  Although drug preparations will usually be carried out by a pharmacist, it is your responsibility to ensure that the instructions are carefully followed.

- Description of any impurities
  Make sure that the toxicological studies were performed using material containing the same impurities at the same level. This can be of particluar importance for biotechnological preparations containing proteins.

In the case of intravenous infusions, compatibility with infusion fluids will have been checked, as well as the potential for precipitation on injection, if the compound is poorly soluble.

The early Phase I, and even Phase II, trials are frequently conducted with experimental formulations that will not be marketed, and may be different from the formulation used in the pre-clinical studies. This may result in differences in bioavailability (and thus tissue exposure and pharmacological response) so you should be aware of this possibility. It is unusual for a sponsoring drug company to repeat any of the pre-clinical studies with a new formulation given only to man, but the two formulations should at least show similar in vitro dissolution characteristics.

The data provided for biotechnology products (e.g. monoclonal antibodies, viral vaccines or somatic cell therapy) are largely similar to those provided for any small molecule. However, there are some additional points you should be aware of. Storage requirements are often more stringent for biotechnology products, as they may be particularly susceptible to degradation in certain temperature, light or humidity conditions, and the shelf-life may be short. The risk of viral contamination is a feature common to all biotechnology products derived from mammalian cell lines, and results, or a confirmatory statement, of virus testing on cells and products may be presented in the CIB. There may also be a statement to confirm that steps have been taken to assure freedom from transmissible spongiform encephalopathies (e.g. Bovine Spongiform Encephalopathy or Creutzfeldt-Jakob Disease). If there is no such statement and you are concerned about such a risk you are advised to discuss this with the sponsoring drug company.

Pre-clinical section

A brief explanation of some of the terminology used in pharmacology sections is presented at the end of this chapter. However, you should refer to some of the standard texts for further information.

Pharmacology

- *In-vitro*

Biochemical experiments are conducted to demonstrate activity, potency and specificity of the study drug. Experiments are carried out on isolated tissue preparations to show the potency, specificity, selectivity, duration of action and tissue concentration–response relationships.

Broad spectrum receptor screens (receptograms) and enzyme screens are used routinely to determine the specificity of the study drug, and studies to investigate interactions with ion channels are also performed.

- *In-vivo*

Experiments on whole animals are performed to investigate the drug's primary pharmacological action in-vivo. Animal models of disease are used to demonstrate the required response, as a prediction of efficacy in humans, and to define the tissue concentration-response relationship. The use of transgenic animals in this area is rapidly expanding.

Whenever possible, a positive control of the same therapeutic class should be used, which can greatly aid dose-selection for the first time in man studies.

You should pay particular attention to:

- The route of administration used (and any discrepancies in response between different routes in the same species)
- The plasma/tissue concentration at which dynamic responses occurred
- The duration of the response
- Evidence of rebound or tachyphylaxis
- Discrepancies in response between species

In vivo whole animal experiments may be performed on a variety of species. It is important to appreciate some general peculiarities of different models. For example, the cardiovascular system in the dog is dominated by vagal tone, and drugs acting on the sympathetic or parasympathetic systems may behave differently in man. Bronchoconstriction in the guinea pig (a species often used for testing anti-asthma drugs) is histamine dependent, whereas histamine plays little or no role in asthma in man.

- Safety pharmacology

Safety pharmacology studies establish the effects of a drug on the major systems of the body, including behavioural responses and cardiovascular, respiratory and gastrointestinal effects. Overt pharmacodynamic effects such as changes in respiration rate and depth, heart rate, and body temperature, and marked vasoconstriction or vasodilatation are measured in conscious animals, usually the mouse and dog, using a range of doses. Evidence of autonomic nervous system or any central effects is also determined.

Further studies in anaesthetised and conscious animals such as rats, dogs or cats determine the cardiovascular and respiratory effects of the drug in more detail. Gastrointestinal motility following oral administration can be studied in mice or rats.

The barbiturate-induced sleeping time is sometimes used as a measure of the effect of the drug on liver metabolism – the sleeping time is reduced if liver enzymes have been induced, and increased if liver enzymes have been inhibited. Primate self-administration studies may be used to assess the abuse potential of centrally-acting drugs, if there is a reason to suspect this.

The observations of a trained and experienced safety pharmacologist can be of considerable help, as they may predict possible effects in man that might warrant more focussed investigations in the human studies.

- Toxicology

There are regulatory requirements for certain toxicological studies to be performed prior to commencing clinical studies and prior to marketing. The International Conference on Harmonisation (ICH) has made great progress in aligning these requirements between Japan, USA and the European Community, but some differences still exist. The rationale of the studies performed and their design should be described in the CIB, and, most importantly, the relevance of the results to human administration at the dose-levels proposed.

The toxicology section of a CIB is usually divided into the following subsections: single dose (acute) toxicity, repeat dose toxicity, carcinogenicity, reproductive toxicity and genotoxicity. Each of these is described below. The toxicology requirements for biotechnology products are described separately.

- Single (acute) and Repeated Dose Toxicology

The objective of this part of the drug development programme is to administer single and repeated doses of the drug at various dose levels to cohorts of animals and observe effects in behaviour, general well-being, major organ function, effects on haematological and biochemical markers. At autopsy, effects on individual organs and tissues are studied using microscopical analyses of tissue sections (histopathology).

The single dose studies define the maximum non-lethal dose (MNLD) in two species (usually rat and mouse), and may identify target organ toxicity. Two routes of administration should be studied – systemic (usually intravenous) and the intended clinical route. If the intended clinical route is intravenous then this route alone is acceptable.

- Repeated dose toxicology

The repeated dose studies are performed in a rodent and a non-rodent (usually rat and dog). Preliminary (dose range finding) studies define the maximum repeatable dose (MRD) in each species. The highest dose administered in the formal repeat dose studies is usually the MRD. Two or three lower doses and a vehicle control are also studied. Plasma drug concentrations are measured in these studies, and pharmacokinetic analyses performed. At the end of each study a proportion of animals demonstrating toxicity are retained for assessment of recovery.

Boxes 3.2 and 3.3 present the required duration of repeated dose studies to support clinical studies and marketing. The first time in man study (using single doses) is usually supported by at least 14 days exposure in the toxicology species. Thereafter, toxicological cover is on a "one to one" ratio with human exposure, (ICH Guidelines M3, non-clinical safety studies for the conduct of human clinical trials for pharmaceuticals).

Occasionally it may be desirable to test a number of similar compounds in man at single doses in order to identify the most appropriate compound to progress. For example, a lead compound may be selected from a group of similar compounds tested in man on the basis of its superior kinetic profile, or superior effect on a surrogate marker. To facilitate this approach, the US Food and Drug Administration (FDA) allows specially designed single dose studies with extended examinations in a rodent and non-rodent to support single dose studies in man (FDA Guidance for Industry PT1, Single dose acute toxicity testing for pharmaceuticals).

As an investigator, you need be assured that these requirements have been met and that the regulatory authority has been informed of the results, as appropriate. What do you need to look for in the results to be satisfied that you can administer the drug for the first time to a human being? The essential points in the single and repeated dose studies are:

Box 3.2 Single and repeated dose toxicity requirements to support Phase I and II studies in the EU and Phase I, II and III studies I the US and Japan.

Duration of clinical trial	Minimum duration of repeated dose toxicity studies	
	Rodents	Non-rodents
Single dose	2 weeks[1] (4 weeks – Japan)	2 weeks
Up to 2 weeks	2 weeks (4 weeks - Japan)	2 weeks
Up to 1 month	1 month	1 month
Up to 3 months	3 months	3 months
Up to 6 months	6 months	6 months
> 6 months	6 months	9 months[2]

[1]In the US, specially designed single dose studies with extended examinations can support single dose clinical studies
[2]Regulatory authorities may request a 12 month study or accept a 6 month study, determined on a case-by-case basis.

Box 3.3 Repeated dose toxicity requirements to support Phase III studies in the EU and marketing in all regions.

Duration of clinical trial	Minimum duration of repeated dose toxicity studies	
	Rodents	Non-rodents
Up to 2 weeks	1 month	1 month
Up to 1 month	3 months	3 months
Up to 3 months	6 months	3 months[1]
> 3 months	6 months	9 months[2]

[1]For marketing, a chronic non-rodent study is recommended if clinical use > 1 month.
[2]Regulatory authorities may request a 12 month study or accept a 6 month study, determined on a case-by-case basis.

- The maximum tolerated dose in the more sensitive species.
- The 'no effect' repeatable dose in the more sensitive species.
- The findings in the concurrent (or historical) controls.
- The number of animals studied in each group and the survival rate, i.e. compare the number that start and finish the experiment
- The tissue exposure at the end of the dosing periods, i.e. the AUC and peak plasma concentration of parent and, if available, active metabolites.

Prediction of safety and tolerability in man based on toxicology studies is notoriously difficult, but you should look for:

- Evidence of adequate tissue exposure to the drug (see below).
- Evidence of satisfactory 'overage' in blood/tissue drug levels between the 'no effect' level in the most sensitive species and the proposed starting and top doses in man. Account must be taken of the absorption, distribution, metabolism and excretion, which may differ between the toxicological species and man.
- Time to onset of the adverse effects
- Duration of effects
- Evidence of recovery of these effects after dosing has ceased.

If a target organ has been identified are there any surrogate markers of toxicity that could be measured in man?

- Toxicokinetics

Measurement of plasma (or serum) concentrations of drug in the animal studies is essential if one is to interpret the safety and pharmacological studies and relate those results to the predicted effects in man. By comparing the drug concentrations required to achieve the desired pharmacological response in the *in-vivo* pharmacology studies with the concentrations associated with unwanted effects in the safety pharmacology and toxicology studies, a therapeutic index can be defined.

Determination of major or active metabolites and their pharmacokinetics is also important. Major metabolites may not have the same activity as the parent drug, but may have other "toxic" properties.

The peak plasma concentration (C_{max}), time to peak concentration and rate of clearance determine total exposure. Bioavailability is a measure of the systemic exposure achieved with the route of administration used, and is an indicator of the likely organ exposure. A large volume of distribution indicates tissue uptake. Evidence of accumulation may be seen in the repeat dose studies, indicating saturation of metabolism, enzyme inhibition, or an intrinsically long half life. Conversely a drop in plasma levels following repeat dosing may indicate enzyme induction.

The variability in the pharmacokinetic parameters is an important factor when considering the desired profile in man. Variable absorption (due to a food effect for example) will lead to unpredictable systemic exposure, which in turn may lead to unpredictable efficacy or side-effects.

Whole body autoradiography quantifies the distribution of the drug, and mass-balance studies determine the disposition of the drug and its metabolites.

In vitro studies determine plasma protein binding in a number of species (including man) over a wide dose-range. Microsomal preparations and individually isolated isozymes are used to identify specific isozymes involved in the metabolism of the drug. Cultured hepatocyte or microsomal preparations are used to screen for cytochrome P450 enzyme induction or inhibition potential, which may support or preclude the need to perform drug interaction studies in humans.

If there are significant gender differences in the pharmacokinetics of the study drug, or any significant differences between species, the CIB should discuss the potential relevance to man.

You should be wary of any direct extrapolation of these data from animals to man. Interspecies scaling is more predictive if several animal species have been evaluated and there is low variability in the metabolic profile of the drug between species. However, you can not exclude the possibility of significant differences in the pharmacokinetics of a drug in man.

- Carcinogenicity (Oncogenicity)

Carcinogenicity studies are designed to assess the potential of the drug to cause neoplastic changes. Not all drugs require carcinogenicity studies, but those likely to be used chronically (3 - 6 months plus) or have frequent intermittent use should be tested (ICH Guidelines S1A, Final guideline on the need for long-term rodent carcinogenicity studies of pharmaceuticals). Likewise those drugs that may give cause for concern (e.g. by virtue of their chemical structure or positive genotoxicity test results) should also be tested. Even in these circumstances, if the life-expectancy of the target patient population is short, long-term carcinogenicity studies may not be required.

The ICH recommends a long-term carcinogenicity in rodents (usually the rat) plus an additional *in vivo* test -

either a short or medium term *in vivo* rodent test system e.g. models of carcinogenesis using neonatal or transgenic mice or a long-term carcinogenicity study in a second rodent species –usually the mouse, (ICH Guidelines S1B, Testing for carcinogenicity of pharmaceuticals).

Carcinogenicity study results are generally required prior to marketing, and would only be completed prior to Phase III trials if there was special concern.

• Reproductive toxicity

These studies investigate the effect of the drug on fertility, reproductive performance, foetal organogenesis, and peri- and post-natal development. Studies should be in mammals, and are usually performed in the rat. In addition, embryo-foetal development studies (which include teratology studies) are conducted in a non-rodent species, usually the rabbit.

The ICH provides guidelines describing the studies required prior to clinical trials (M3, Nonclinical safety studies for the conduct of human clinical trials for pharmaceuticals), and those required prior to marketing (S5A, Detection of toxicity to reproduction for medicinal products and S5B, Addendum on toxicity to male fertility). Since evaluation of the reproductive organs is performed in the repeat dose studies, males and sterilised or post-menopausal females may be included in Phase I and II trials prior to reproduction toxicity studies. A male fertility study should be completed prior to the initiation of Phase III trials.

In Japan, female fertility and embryo-foetal development studies in animals are required before any study using female subjects of child bearing potential (but using effective contraception). In the EU embryo-foetal development assessment is required prior to Phases I and II, and female fertility assessment is required prior to Phase III. In the US, females of childbearing potential may be included in early trials without reproduction toxicity studies in animals as long as certain precautions are taken. These include appropriate contraception, frequent pregnancy testing, and entry after a confirmed menstrual period. Both female fertility and embryo-foetal development studies are required prior to Phase III.

- Genotoxicity

Genotoxicity tests are designed to identify compounds that may induce genetic damage. A standard battery of tests is described by the ICH (S2B Genotoxicity: A standard battery for genotoxicity testing of pharmaceuticals).

- A test for gene mutation in bacteria (e.g. Ames test)
- An in vitro test with cytogenetic evaluation of chromosomal damage with mammalian cells or an in vitro mouse lymphoma thymidine kinase (tk) assay
- An in vivo test for chromosomal damage using rodent haemopoetic cells

This approach is designed to reduce the risk of false negative results for compounds with genotoxic potential, and a single positive result in one of the tests does not necessarily mean that the test compound poses a genotoxic risk to humans.

Usually the first two tests will be performed prior to human exposure, but the full battery must be completed prior to Phase II studies. If indicated, additional genotoxicity tests may be performed.

Toxicology testing of biotechnology-derived pharmaceuticals

The standard regime of toxicology studies for mainstream pharmaceutical products is generally not appropriate for biotechnology- derived drugs (biopharmaceuticals) (see ICH Guidelines S6, Preclinical safety evaluation of biotechnology-derived pharmaceuticals). The choice of species used in the toxicology studies will depend on expression of the relevant receptor (or epitope in the case of monoclonal antibodies). If no relevant species exist, homologous proteins or transgenic animals expressing the human receptor may be studied. You should check that the product used in the toxicology studies is of comparable purity, stability and potency to the clinical supplies you will receive. Specific studies may have been performed to demonstrate this.

Single and repeated dose studies are required, but additional immunological studies are important in order to aid interpretation of the repeated dose studies, since biotechnology products intended for humans may elicit an immune response in the animals tested. Such antibody responses may affect the PK/PD parameters or adverse event profile, but should not affect the interpretation of the repeated dose studies unless they significantly alter the pharmacological or toxicological effects of the product. Reproductive studies specifically designed to assess developmental immunotoxicity may be required, on a case by case basis.

The standard battery of genotoxicity studies is not appropriate for biotechnology products (although specific studies may be performed if there is cause for concern about the product e.g. if an organic linker molecule is present in a conjugate protein product) Similarly, standard carcinogenicity studies are not generally appropriate for biotechnology products, but long-term rodent studies may be performed in certain circumstances e.g. if the compound has the potential to induce cell proliferation, (ICH Guidelines S1A, The need for long-term rodent carcinogenicity studies of pharmaceuticals).

Clinical section

Obviously the amount of clinical data you will have to review will depend on the stage of development of the study drug. For the first administration of the drug to man, you will only have the preclinical data, plus any available data on human exposure to drugs of the same or similar class. Alternatively a study in Phase III or IV may have supporting data from several thousands of patients.

Clinical Pharmacology

Tolerability and safety

Whatever the stage of drug development, it is crucial that you know the complete safety and tolerability profile of the drug in all patients studied, even if some of the data are preliminary.

Tolerability and safety data are collected by recording all adverse events, measurement of laboratory safety measures (blood biochemistry, haematology and urinalysis) and other dynamic measures (e.g. 12 lead electrocardiograms, blood pressure, pulse rate).

Most drug-related adverse events in Phase I trials are predictable, dose-related and due to the known pharmacological effect of the drug (e.g. bradycardia with b-blockers). However, adverse events may be seen at lower than expected doses if the tissue-receptor concentration of the drug is greater than predicted from animal studies. This can be due to better drug absorption in man, better tissue transfer (e.g. across the blood-brain barrier), different distribution of specific receptors or presence of active metabolites not seen in animals.

Adverse events may occur if the drug is less specific in its action than predicted from animal studies (e.g. a different receptor class is antagonised or stimulated), or if the drug is less selective in its action than predicted from animal studies (e.g. a different sub-class of the specific receptor is antagonised or stimulated).

Idiosyncratic adverse drug reactions are much less common but may still be detected in early phase studies. These would not be expected from the known pharmacology of the drug, and may be due to an immunological reaction, or an inherited abnormality of the subject (e.g. a genetic polymorphism affecting the metabolic pathway of the drug).

Attributing causality of adverse events to study drug can be extremely difficult with the limited exposure during Phase I. A significant proportion of adverse events reported in Phase I trials could be related to study conditions – for example fasting or caffeine withdrawal. However, you should maintain a low threshold for suspecting that adverse events could be drug-related.

When reviewing adverse event data you should determine:

- The number of subjects in whom a particular event was reported, compared with the number exposed
- The dose at which the event occurred, and the route of administration
- The time to onset, course and exact description of the event
- The clinical management (and antidote if appropriate)
- The effect of re-challenge, if performed
- The "no-effect" dose

Non-serious adverse events are summarised in the CIB, often in tabular form. A serious adverse event is defined as "Any untoward medical occurrence that at any dose results in death, is life-threatening, requires in-patient hospitalisation or prolongation of existing hospitalisation, results in persistent or significant disability/incapacity or a congenital anomaly/birth defect." Some Regulatory Authorities also include cancer and overdose in this definition. Serious adverse events are described in more detail (usually individually) in the text of the CIB.

When interpreting adverse event data, beware of pooling of data from studies with different designs (e.g. open versus double-blind, placebo-controlled). Look out for patterns of events in sub-groups of subjects – prevalence in one sex or ethnic group, or those taking a particular concomitant medication for example. Determine the temporal relationship of adverse events to dosing – does this correlate with the plasma concentration of the drug or metabolite? Did the adverse event end when the dosing was ended, or soon afterwards? Did the adverse event start prior to drug administration, and if so, was it exacerbated by drug exposure?

The number of dropouts in a study is often a clue to the tolerability of the study drug, even if adverse events are not reported. Look at the proportion of subjects on active treatment who withdraw, compared with the number on placebo.

You need to be reassured that you are not putting your trial population at undue risk. A direct discussion with the drug company physician responsible for the programme is very useful, and frequently allays anxiety. You should ascertain whether any special tests or monitoring procedures should be included in future studies, or whether certain sub-populations of subjects should be excluded from the study population (e.g. slow metabolisers).

- Laboratory safety tests

Laboratory safety tests (standard haematological and biochemical investigations) are routinely performed before, during and after drug exposure. Additional tests may be performed to confirm or refute toxicological findings, or to investigate particular pharmacological effects of the drug.

If there are significant abnormalities these will be recorded as adverse events. Even if there are no significant changes look for any trends in one or more parameter. These may remain within the normal range, but could be an indication of an underlying toxicity. Are there clusters of investigations that are abnormal (e.g. liver function tests or white cell counts) that may indicate specific drug toxicity? Were all abnormalities followed up until resolution?

As with adverse event data, look for any link between

the abnormality and subject subgroups, and consider any pertinent additional tests to include at screening or during the study.

- Pharmacodynamics

Some pharmacodynamic measures (e.g. ECG, blood pressure and heart rate) are often included as part of the safety and tolerability measurements in early trials. These and other dynamic data collected can be of great value to the investigator for:

- Confirmation of the biological hypothesis in man.
- Construction of a dose-response curve
- Justification of selection of doses for further study
- Calculation of the therapeutic index

It is also useful to correlate the dynamic response with pharmacokinetic parameters with the aim to define a pharmacokinetic/pharmacodynamic relationship. The terms used for these measurements have recently been defined by a working group from the US National Institutes of Health.

The decision of which doses to progress into Phase II may rest heavily on the results of certain pharmacodynamic tests used as **biological markers** or **biomarkers**. These are defined as characteristics that are measured and evaluated as an indicator of normal biologic processes, pathogenic processes or pharmacologic responses to a therapeutic intervention. A biomarker has no direct relevance to the **clinical endpoint**, which is simply defined by how a patient feels, functions or survives. **Surrogate markers** are biomarkers that have been validated to substitute for a clinical endpoint.

The term biomarker in this context refers to the use of a clinical or investigational measurement as a proxy for the ultimate clinical endpoint in order to reach an earlier decision point. That is, the biomarker is used as a provision of confidence, rather than a true surrogate of efficacy that could be used to foreshorten a long clinical trial. For example, in a healthy volunteer study with a new anti-platelet agent, bleeding times and ex-vivo platelet aggregration tests may be used for dose-selection, yet there are few data correlating specific levels of platelet inhibition with either efficacy or safety clinical endpoints in patients (Harrington et al 1998).

Disease models in healthy volunteers can be used to confirm the desired pharmacological action in man and may also aid dose-selection, particularly if a dose-response relationship can be well defined. For example ipecacuanha-induced vomiting in healthy subjects was used successfully as a model to test the anti-emetic properties of ondansetron (Minton et al 1993).

- Pharmacokinetics

Depending on the stage of development of the study drug, pharmacokinetic data following single doses over a wide dose range and repeat doses at two to three doses may be available. In addition, interaction studies (with other medications and/or food) and studies in different populations may have been performed. Mass-balance studies using radiolabelled compound will determine the extent to which the parent compound is metabolised, and the predominant route of excretion.

The parameters you should expect to see described are:

- Maximum observed concentration (C_{max}) and time to maximum observed concentration (t_{max})
- Area under the curve (AUC)
- Clearance (CL)
- Terminal/elimination half-life ($t_{1/2}$)
- Volume of distribution (V_d)
- In the case of orally administered compounds the bioavailability (F)

In addition, the presence and pharmacokinetics of active metabolites should be described.

The half-life of the drug (and any active metabolites) will normally determine the dosing regimen of the drug (although this will also depend on the duration of dynamic effects of the drug). These factors will also determine the minimum washout period between treatment periods in a cross-over design study.

The volume of distribution of a drug is largely determined by its lipophilicity. A lipophilic drug will be expected to have a large V_d, and to cross the blood brain barrier readily. In contrast, a highly polar drug is likely to be restricted to the vascular compartment, and will have a small V_d. The degree of plasma protein binding will be determined from in vitro studies, but if highly bound the potential for significant drug-drug interactions due to displacement from plasma proteins may be more of a theoretical than real risk (Rolan, 1994)

Absolute bioavailability will only be quoted if a study has been performed comparing intravenous administration with the route of administration in question (usually oral). However, relative bioavailability between different formulations may be given. Large variability in bioavailability can be due to a number of factors, including variable release rates from the formulation, effect of pH on disintegration of the formulation and absorption of active components, effects of food and high "first-pass" metabolism through the gut wall and liver. Enterohepatic recirculation (excretion of the drug via the bile into the small intestine, followed by reabsorption into the hepatic portal vein) will prolong the systemic exposure to the drug.

A greater than proportional increase of C_{max} and AUC across ascending doses may give an indication of saturation of clearance mechanisms, which in turn may lead to accumulation of study drug or its metabolites in the repeat dose studies.

Mass-balance studies using radiolabelled compound will determine the extent to which the parent compound is metabolised, and the predominant route of excretion. Can all or most of the administered dose be accounted for in the urine and faeces?

Look for differences in each of the pharmacokinetic parameters in sub-groups of the population studied; are there any sex or age differences for example? Do any concomitant medications result in an altered pharmacokinetic profile of the drug? At a later stage of drug development these answers may be available from population pharmacokinetic analyses, using limited samples from patients in large scale Phase III trials.

Finally, look at the inter-subject variability in the pharmacokinetic parameters. Are the data skewed by outliers? Will it be difficult to predict exposure following a given dose? This is particularly important if the drug has a narrow therapeutic index. If this is a concern, and variability data are not given in the CIB, you should ask the sponsoring drug company representatives for this data.

- Imaging

The use of imaging in drug development is becoming more and more common. The time-course and extent of tissue delivery of radio-labelled drugs can be measured using gamma-scintigraphy, positron emission tomography (PET) or single photon computerised tomography (SPECT), for example. PET can also be used to localise receptor binding, and receptor occupancy can be quantified using displacement techniques, and dose-occupancy curves generated. If the level of receptor occupancy correlates with efficacy endpoints, then this could be used for dose-selection. The duration of receptor occupancy may determine the frequency of dose administration, and length of washout period. The cerebral pharmacokinetics of a centrally-acting drug can be derived from such studies, and may be quoted in the CIB to justify dose-selection and dosing regimens.

Subtle structural changes in organs can be measured using magnetic resonance imaging (MRI) and the effect of drugs on these changes (e.g. slowing of brain atrophy in a chronic neurodegenerative disorder, or shrinkage of a tumour, or infarct lesion) can be used as efficacy endpoints, or more strictly speaking, biomarkers.

Functional imaging (PET, SPECT or fMRI) can be used to localise and quantify effects of the drug on the metabolic activity of tissues (e.g. altered regional cerebral blood flow or cerebral glucose metabolism). This may demonstrate effect of the drug in areas other than the primary site of action, and may help to explain an adverse event for example.

- Risk groups and drug interactions

Specific studies are performed to investigate the safety, pharmacodynamics and pharmacokinetics of the study drug when given in combination with another drug, or when administered to a subject in a risk group (e.g. hepatically or renally-impaired patients, or the elderly).

There should be a theoretical rationale why such a study is needed (e.g. high first pass metabolism of a drug could justify a specific study in patients with liver failure). Animal data or in vitro data using human tissues (e.g. isolated liver microsomes or liver slices) may provide further indication that a study in man is required.

Pharmacokinetic and dynamic interactions may achieve statistical significance but do not necessarily have any clinical consequence, and you may have to balance this if including "at-risk" patients in the study population.

The CIB should provide details of contraindications, warnings and precautions, with guidance on the use of the study drug in situations in which no clinical data are currently available (e.g. pregnancy, breast-feeding, children etc.). Any evidence for abuse and/or dependence potential should be described, and information about the management of overdose (including antidote instructions) should be included in the CIB.

- Clinical trials

At the later stages of drug development more information on patients will be available. What you need to establish from this section of the CIB will depend on the precise study you are being asked to conduct. Usually by this stage safety and tolerability of the study drug are less of an issue than in the early phases. The information presented in the CIB should be sufficient to justify the duration and range of doses you are being asked to study.

Evidence of efficacy in later patient studies is provided by the results of placebo and active comparator controlled trials. Details of the designs of the trials, outcome measures and the populations studied should be provided in the CIB. Look for any variables that might have affected an efficacy outcome.

At this stage, genotyping may have been performed on the trial population, and a relationship between a certain genotype and an efficacy or safety endpoint may have been found. If this is the case you may have to pre-screen your trial subjects in order to exclude or include subjects on the basis of their genotype, or you may be asked to collect DNA samples for future analysis. If you are asked to do this, ensure that both you and the sponsoring drug company are fully aware of your ethical and legal responsibilities in terms of patient consent, analysis, storage and destruction of the samples, confidentiality of data and returning results to the patients.

Summary The main points that you should seek in the CIB, or from the sponsoring drug company's representative are:

- Data supporting the quality of the pharmaceutical product, in the formulation to be used
- Evidence that the study drug has the desired pharmacological effect
- Evidence that the appropriate toxicological studies for the population to be studied and the stage of development have been performed
- Demonstration of adequate tissue exposure in the toxicology species used
- A summary of all human exposure, with safety, dynamic, kinetic and efficacy results
- Justification for the dose selection and dosing regimen
- A list of actual and theoretical risks associated with the administration of the study drug.
- Approval from the appropriate Regulatory Authority where necessary.

Definitions of pharmacological terms

Agonist
A signalling molecule (hormone neurotransmitter or synthetic drug) that binds to a receptor and activates it by inducing a conformational change, which produces a pharmacological response, e.g. muscle contraction or relaxation, secretion, change in enzyme activity etc.

Antagonist
This is a drug that attenuates the effect of an agonist. It may be competitive (or surmountable) i.e. binds reversibly to a region of the receptor which overlaps with the binding site for the agonist, but occupies the site without activating the effector mechanism. Non-competitive (insurmountable) antagonism is said to be present when no amount of agonist can completely overcome the inhibition once it is established (unlike competitive antagonism).

Potency
A measure of the concentrations of a drug at which it is effective. It is a vague term and should always be further defined.

For agonists, the terms of definitions used include:

- EC_{50} - is the molar concentration of an agonist which produces 50% of the maximum possible response for that agonist. Sometimes other percentage values are used (EC_{25}, EC_{40}, etc).

- IC_{50} - where an agonist causes an inhibitory response, the IC_{50} is the molar concentration which produces 50% of its maximum possible inhibition. For these two measures a lower value indicates higher potency.

For antagonists, further definition of potency is frequently given by one or more of the following terms:

- PA_2 - is a logarithmic measure and is the negative log of the concentration of antagonist which would produce a twofold shift in the concentration-response curve for an agonist. A higher value denotes greater potency.
- K_B - is the equilibrium dissociation constant for a competitive antagonist, the concentration which would occupy 50% of the receptors at equilibrium.
- PK_B - is a measure of the potency of a competitive antagonist; it is the negative log of the molar concentration which at equilibrium would occupy 50% of the receptor in the absence of agonist.

Efficacy

Not to be confused with clinical efficacy, this describes the way in which agonists vary in the response they produce, even when they occupy the same number of receptors. High-efficacy agonists can produce their maximal response whilst occupying a relatively low proportion of receptors; lower-efficacy agonists may not be able to produce the same maximum response even when occupying the entire receptor population.

Figure 3.1 A response vs log concentration curve for two agonists. Drug B is more potent than Drug A, but has lower efficacy. Log EC50 values are shown

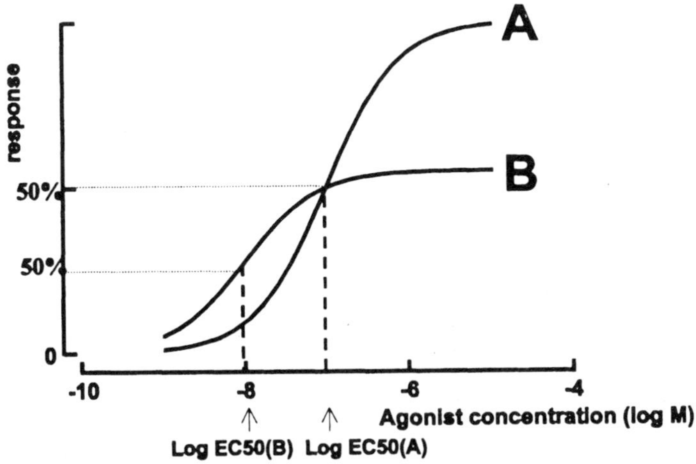

Figure 3.2 Potency of a competitive agonist. Idealised concentration curves fo an agonist under control conditions (curve A) and in the presence of two concentrations of a competitive antagonist (curves B and C). Note that a competitive agonist does not depress the maximum response to the agonist.
Reproduced with kind permission of Dr M.J Sheehan

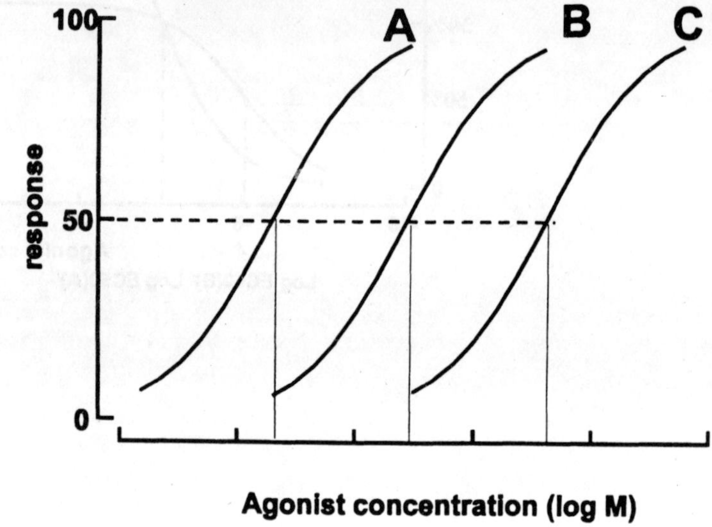

References

- Harrington RA, Kleiman NS, Granger CB, et al. Relation between inhibition of platelet aggregation and clinical outcomes. Am Heart J 1998; 136: S43-S50.
- Minton N, Swift R, Lawlor C et al. Ipecacuanha-induced emesis: a human model for testing antiemetic drug activity. Clin Pharm Ther 1993; 54: 53-57.
- Rolan PE. Plasma protein binding displacement interactions – why are they still regarded as clinically important? Br J Clin Pharm 1994; 37, 125-128.

Useful Websites

- International Conference on Harmonisation (ICH) *http://www.pharmweb.net/pwmirror/pw9/ifpma/ich1.html*

- FDA Guidance pages
  http://www.fda.gov/cder/guidance/index.htm
  On this website you can access all documents on drug development issued by the US Food and Drug Administration.
- The European Agency for the Evaluation of Medicinal Products
  http://www.eudra.org/en_home.htm
  This website provides access to the full text of all regulatory guidelines in addition to other useful guidelines issued by the European Medicines Agency. This includes the ICH documents - which can also be found on the FDA site.

Further Reading

- Rang H.P. and Dale M.M. (1995). Pharmacology. Edinburgh: Churchill Livingstone.
- Sheehan M (1999). Pocket Guide to Pharmacology. Available from: Educational Liaison, Glaxo Wellcome Medicines Research Centre, Gunnels Wood Road, Stevenage, Hertfordshire, UK. SG1 2NY.
- Griffin J. P., O'Grady J, D'Arcy P.F. (1998). Textbook of Pharmaceutical Medicine. Queen's University of Belfast.

4

The first administration of a new active substance to humans

John Posner

Introduction

The first administration of a new chemical or biological substance to humans may be conducted in a Phase I unit of a pharmaceutical company or contract research organisation (CRO) or in a hospital by an academic investigator. There has been an expansion of all such activities in recent years and the whole Phase I area has been put on a much more professional footing. To some extent the setting depends on whether the volunteers are healthy or patients since patients are generally more accessible in hospitals whilst CROs tend to use healthy volunteers. Whatever the setting and the nature of the volunteers, there are special considerations which pertain to all such studies. The same considerations are relevant to many studies performed at an early stage of a drug's development not only to the first administration. Thus, academic researchers frequently find themselves being asked by pharmaceutical companies to administer doses that are higher than studied hitherto or to study a drug in a population which might be much more susceptible to adverse reactions than young healthy volunteers or in circumstances where it will be much more difficult to keep the volunteers under close observation. Some of the particular points pertaining to such studies will be discussed in this chapter.

What do you need to know about the drug?

This question is addressed in detail in Chapter 3 and will be summarised briefly here with discussion of one or two points which need to be emphasised. Before contemplating administration of any new active substance to a human, you need to have detailed information about the following:

Preclinical evaluation

- Toxicology and mutagenicity
- Primary and secondary pharmacological activity in

animals
- Pharmacokinetics and metabolism in animals
- Sensitivity and specificity of assays of parent drug and metabolites
- Chemistry, physical properties, pharmaceutics

Clinical evaluation (if studies have been performed)
- Tolerability (with a listing of all adverse events whether or not they are considered likely to be drug related)
- Any evidence of pharmacodynamic activity or efficacy
- Pharmacokinetics and metabolism

Although there are clear regulatory guidelines (see Chapter 3) which can help one verify that appropriate toxicity studies have been carried out to support the proposed dosing period in humans (summarised in Chapter 3), there are no simple formulae for interpreting preclinical data. Essentially, one needs to go through a two-stage process:

- Based on the primary pharmacology in animals, what doses and, more importantly, what exposure to drug is likely to be necessary to achieve the desired therapeutic effect?
- Can the doses that produce this desired exposure to drug and its metabolites be supported in man by the toxicology and secondary pharmacology in animals?

There are no simple answers when it comes to deciding what is a reasonable margin of safety; this will very much depend on the steepness of the dose response curve for pharmacodynamic effects and just what those effects are. For example, one would be very concerned if ventricular arrhythmias were seen in animals at plasma concentrations just above those likely to be therapeutic which proved fatal in most animals after a small dose increment. By contrast, a small dose-related reduction of blood pressure starting at the high end of the putative therapeutic range of concentration which increased by 5% for each doubling of dose in anaesthetised animals would be of far less concern. Similarly, our approach to organ toxicity must be considered on a case by case basis, taking into account the nature of the toxicity observed as well as the relative exposure to drug and metabolites.

It is possible that the preclinical safety data give no

cause for concern and it is clear that they are quite sufficient to support the proposed human exposure. On the other hand, careful scrutiny of the data may suggest that the dosing regimen originally intended will have to be modified or even that is unsafe to proceed without further information. Such decisions often require fine judgement based on a combination of medical common sense, experience of dealing with toxicological issues as well as a knowledge of the specific drug class. If in doubt, don't rely on an Ethics Committee to make the decision for you; ask to speak to a senior toxicologist of the company and if you need further reassurance after that, seek an independent expert opinion having first agreed this with the company and made arrangements for confidentiality to be maintained.

Study objectives

It should not be necessary to state that every study must have clear objectives and that the design of the study must enable those objectives to be met but sadly, it is all too common for neither of these conditions to be satisfied. So called 'pilot studies' in early drug development frequently have very vague objectives eg 'to obtain some preliminary information on efficacy and safety'. Numbers of subjects are often far too small to provide sufficient statistical power and controls for comparison may be inadequate or non-existent. When there are such fundamental deficiencies, it is entirely predictable that the results will at best be difficult to interpret and at worst may be quite useless. Certainly, they are highly unlikely to be sufficiently reliable to form the basis for crucial decisions such as establishing the doses to be used in forthcoming large clinical trials or whether to stop drug development forthwith. The amount of effort taken to perform a poor study is no less and often greater than one with explicit objectives and a scientifically robust design and of course such unsatisfactory experimentation is also unethical.

Here are some specific objectives that are fairly typical of early studies in man with a new active substance:

- To investigate the tolerability and pharmacokinetics of intravenous infusions of Drug X administered for 1 hour in a range of doses (increments and range need to be specified) to healthy young volunteers.
- To investigate tolerability and determine steady state plasma concentrations and characterise the

pharmacokinetics of Drug X and its major metabolites when Drug X is administered orally in a dose of y mg twice daily for 7 days to healthy elderly volunteers.

- To investigate the relationship between dose, plasma concentration and inhibition of Enzyme Y with single doses of Drug X administered to patients with asthma of mild or moderate severity.
- To establish the maximum tolerated dose and plasma concentrations of the cytotoxic drug X in patients with Stage IV carcinoma of the colon.

Note that each objective is quite specific even though there may be very little or no prior information about how the drug behaves in man. It is frequently possible to satisfy a number of objectives eg pharmacokinetics, tolerability and a pharmacodynamic measure but it is important to define which are primary. Information about secondary objectives may be valuable but it should be recognised from the outset that they will need further elucidation in later studies. The study must be designed to meet the primary objectives and it doesn't pay to be too greedy. There are simple practical constraints which need to be recognised. It may seem reasonable to record a 12 lead electrocardiogram, take a blood sample and have the volunteer perform a psychometric test simultaneously but the chances are that the quality of the electrocardiogram will be poor due to muscle movement artefact and chest leads falling off, the blood sample won't be taken on time and performance of the psychometric task will be very variable because the subject is disturbed by the other procedures. It may be possible to schedule all these procedures sensibly but there is a limit to what can be achieved without compromising the quality of data collected.

Having listed the study objectives, it is worth standing back from the detail to ask oneself what contribution the study will make to development of the drug. If everything goes to plan, will the results contribute to establishing the appropriate dose range for large trials of efficacy and safety? Are they likely to verify that the pharmacodynamic activity predicted from studies with various plasma concentrations in animals is seen in similar concentrations in man? Will the data generated in healthy volunteers be relevant to future studies in patients? While it is frequently unrealistic to expect a single study to provide all the answers, there is no justification for proceeding with the planned study if there is real doubt that it will progress the drug's development.

Aspects of study design

Assessment of tolerability

Tolerability is almost always one of the primary objectives of the first or subsequent studies in man. This needs to be explored over a range of doses generally using a dose-escalating design. The relevance of the data can only be interpreted in the context of plasma concentrations thought to be in the therapeutic range and/or measures of pharmacodynamic activity which may serve as biomarkers or surrogates and are presumed to be predictive of therapeutic efficacy. Clearly the absence of adverse events at plasma concentrations which are one tenth those required for therapeutic effect is little reassurance and the presence of adverse events at concentrations ten times higher than those required may not pose any problem.

There are several parameters of interest in assessing tolerability of any drug. These may include symptomatology and vital signs such as heart rate and blood pressure or measures such as ST segments or QT intervals on an electrocardiogram. Laboratory assessments such as white cell and platelet counts, coagulation tests and renal and liver function tests also fall into this category and may actually constitute sought endpoints eg evidence of myelosuppression with a cytotoxic agent.

Many of these are standard clinical procedures but the collection of symptoms in early drug studies merits some discussion because reliance on spontaneous reporting is generally unsatisfactory. Every symptom reported should be recorded separately and for each symptom one needs to know its maximum severity, duration and whether any action was required. In order to capture duration, the time of onset and termination need to be known but most of us only have a vague idea of when for example a headache actually started and finished even if we are reporting the symptom on the day it occurred. It is therefore better to actively seek adverse events by interrogating the subject at intervals which need to be specified in the protocol. Typically this needs to be frequent in the first few hours after drug administration and then at progressively wider spaced intervals later in the day and during the follow up period. There then arises the question of the best way to actively elicit symptoms. One possibility is to administer a check list of about 20 symptoms each time which might include symptoms which are expected from what is known about the drug and others that serve as 'fillers' which could occur but are not expected. There must of course be the opportunity to report and rate symptoms not listed as well. The problem with the check list approach is that before (too long) one has a list of 15 different complaints reported by several subjects on a number of occasions due to suggestibility and it soon becomes extremely difficult to establish which are likely to be attributable to drug and which are not. An alternative approach is to ask a standard open question at specified times after drug administration. The wording needs to be simple and without any element of suggestion leaving the subject to report any symptoms or not as they feel. An example of such a question is:

Do you feel unwell or different from usual in any way?

The answer is 'Yes' or 'No' and this response must be recorded on the case report form. If the response is 'Yes', the symptom, its severity, time and likely attributability (in the judgement of the investigator) need to be recorded on a separate form, an example of which is shown in Figure 4.1. If the symptom has already been reported and is still on going, this is noted and when that symptom is no longer reported the offset time is recorded and hence its total duration determined.

If a symptom requires action to be taken, which might be something quite inconsequential, like 1000mg paracetamol administered for a headache, this must be recorded and of course if the event is more serious, full details need to be documented. In the event of a serious adverse experience which is defined as life threatening or one requiring hospitalisation, this must be reported immediately to the sponsoring pharmaceutical company or other body so that regulatory bodies and other investigators can be informed.

Pharmacodynamics A pharmaceutical company or other institution responsible for the discovery of a drug may approach a particular academic department or individual because they have specialist facilities, interest and expertise in a clinical or research technique. The sponsor will want these skills with a particular methodology to be applied to their drug because it will serve as a direct or surrogate measure of efficacy. A wise investigator will, however, appreciate the limitations of a technique which may be very novel and therefore inadequately validated. It may be well tried and tested for detecting clinical abnormalities but may never have been used for detection of drug effects. There may be little or no information on reproducibility within an individual when the test is performed on different days making it impossible to perform a power calculation. Diurnal changes in a measurement may be unknown and so on. The time to find out the limitations of a technique is *not* when a new drug is being tested for the first time. Methods employed to assess pharmacodynamic effects of new drugs should be fully validated before this and all the practical issues sorted out well in advance too. Simple considerations such as the number of subjects that can be studied on one day because of the time taken to perform a test or the number of samples that can be handled at one time need to be agreed well in advance.

How should the dose be escalated?

For the first administration to humans, the starting dose should generally be a small fraction of the maximum no effect dose in animal toxicity studies (see Box 4.1). There are no simple formulae for this though various attempts have been made to develop such rules. The process for deciding what the dose range should be, is identical to that described above when considering the preclinical and clinical information available to date. However, there is frequently more discussion about the number of dose increments and speed of escalation than the starting dose. Traditionally, doubling increments are employed because biological responses are generally related to dose in a logarithmic fashion and doubling simply provides evenly spaced increments on a $\log_2$ scale. However, in absolute terms, the dose increment from 200 to 400 mg is 10 times greater than that of 20 to 40 mg and it is often prudent to reduce the increments to linear rather than doubling at the higher end, e.g. 100, 200, 300, and 400 mg. If the drug is known to combine with its receptor in a stoichiometric fashion or if the dose response curve is likely to steep, linear increments might be advisable from the outset. The number of such increments will often be limited by practical considerations such as the number of occasions volunteers are available to attend, the duration of the study and the amount of blood loss. Ideally, the number of dose increments should be no more than 6 or 7 so that the study can be conducted in a single group of subjects generally dosed at weekly intervals. However the dosing intervals may need to be lengthened if the half-life of the drug or that of a major metabolite is longer than 24 hours to allow for complete elimination between successive doses. If the dose range to be covered is large and this can only be achieved by 9 or 10 increments, it may be sensible to use two cohorts of subjects, with each cohort receiving alternate doses or with the second cohort starting when the first has completed but with some overlap of doses. The alternating approach has the advantage that no individual is exposed to relatively high doses before having received low ones and pharmacokinetic and pharmacodynamic data are available for each subject over virtually the whole dose range. Remember that a number of approaches are possible and that the most appropriate design for a study must be determined on a case-by-case basis.

Is it necessary to establish a maximum tolerated dose?

Some drugs have a low therapeutic index and the greatest therapeutic benefit will be obtained if administered at a dose which is only slightly less that which causes unacceptable adverse effects. The majority of cytotoxic agents fall into this category as do aminoglycoside antibiotics but the decision to halt a dose-escalation because of adverse effects is not always straightforward. The adverse effects may not be serious but may be disliked by the volunteers. Only physicians can decide whether to continue or stop a study but the investigator is well advised to listen carefully to what volunteers and nursing staff have to say. When hitherto sensible, well motivated volunteers begin to adopt a negative attitude to a study for whatever reason, it is probably time to stop.

By contrast, it is almost impossible to attain the maximum tolerated dose of some drugs eg penicillins and it may be quite unethical to dose deliberately to toxicity. The proponents of this approach have often been guilty of not including any pharmacodynamic assessments or measurement of plasma drug concentrations during the course of the study. For most drugs with a large therapeutic index it is perfectly reasonable to stop dose-escalation when doses required to achieve an endpoint such as complete inhibition of a target enzyme

Box 4.1 Considerations in deciding the starting dose

- Maximum no-effect dose or daily steady state concentrations and AUC in toxicity studies in the most sensitive species
- The nature and severity of behavioural and organ toxicity in animals
- The dose at the lower end of a relevant dose-reponse curve and the slope of the curve
- The pharmacokinetics of parent drug and metabolites in different animal species with particular attention to active metabolites with long half-lives
- The likely range of doses and the number of incremental steps likely to be required to reach the projected top dose

activity or gastric acid secretion have been exceeded. For drugs devoid of pharmacological activity such as antibiotics it is usually justified to stop escalation when a target plasma concentration has been exceeded by a pre-agreed margin. As with animal toxicology, the nature of any toxicity also needs to be considered on a case by case basis and of course the particular disease to be treated forms partof the risk-benefit equation.

Is a placebo group necessary?

If the objectives of the study are restricted to assessments of tolerability and pharmacokinetics, the necessity for a placebo group may seem questionable. It is certainly true that when an active drug produces an obvious effect such as a profound fall in blood pressure or gross central effects, there is no point in trying to perform any statistical comparison between groups and in any case the study has been unblinded. However, what one really wants to know is the tolerability at drug doses which do not produce gross adverse effects. It may be impossible to distinguish small falls in blood pressure or mild sedation or for that matter complaints of headache or nasal stuffiness from symptoms which occur to most volunteers at one time or another under study conditions. Intercurrent viral epidemics, food poisoning and other unpredictable factors often confound studies and interpretation of haematology and clinical chemistry abnormal values may be aided by the presence of a group who did not receive active drug. In general then, first administrations to man should be controlled with a placebo group.

Parallel groups or cross over?

The question of the optimum design then arises and in particular whether to use parallel groups or a cross over design. A typical design involving parallel groups would be to administer single escalating doses of active drug to a group of 12 subjects and matching placebo to another group of 6 or 12, the subjects having been randomly allocated to the active or placebo groups at trial entry ie when they receive their subject numbers. The alternative crossover design might involve 12 or 16 subjects who receive escalating doses but on at least one occasion they are randomised to receive placebo. The dose of active drug which they would have received on that occasion might be omitted ie they skip a dose, or they can receive it on the following occasion so that every subject receives each dose. If placebo is to be administered on more than one occasion, these should not be consecutive occasions for an individual subject.

Thus on each occasion, 8 of 16 subjects might receive active and 8 placebo. If it is felt to be important that every subject receive every dose, the parallel groups design has some advantage as it is completed more quickly ie without interspersed placebo occasions and, if blood is being sampled for pharmacokinetics, with lower total blood loss. However, it often becomes obvious which group is receiving active drug so that the blind is broken for the rest of the study. Comparison of effects between parallel groups are 'between-subject' which is almost always more variable than 'within subject' and therefore lack statistical power. Conversely, it is much easier to maintain the blind throughout the study with the crossover design, it is more economical on numbers of volunteers and has higher statistical power. The usual objections to crossover designs discussed in Chapter 7 which apply to large scale clinical trials in patient populations over long periods do not really apply to these small clinical pharmacology studies.

How many subjects?

Some examples of group size with the two designs are given above but the exact numbers need to be considered carefully for each study. If primary objective of the study is to establish the dose which produces a change of defined magnitude in a specific pharmacodynamic measure eg fall in blood pressure or change in a lung function test, then a power calculation should be performed using variability obtained in previous studies ideally conducted by yourself under the same conditions or, as second best using data from the work of others published in the scientific literature. If, on the other hand, no such measure is to be employed, the number is arrived at empirically. There is no correct number but there has to be a balance between the minimum number on which it is reasonable to base decisions about dose-escalation and the number that it is reasonable to expose to the potential hazards of a new chemical entity. Thus, 4 would almost always be too few and 100 too many. Generally a reasonable number lies somewhere between 12 and 30 but this will be influenced by the number of doses that any individual can receive, the amount of blood to be taken on each occasion, the number of dose increments anticipated and how long it will take to complete the study.

The study population: healthy volunteers or patients?

A healthy volunteer may be defined as 'an individual who is in good general health, not having any mental or physical disorder requiring regular or frequent medication and who is able to give valid informed consent to participation in a study'. For legal reasons, the lower age limit is generally 18 years and the upper is usually 35 or 40 though it may be appropriate to study a population of healthy elderly usually defined as over 64 years even at an early stage of drug development though not generally in the first study. They may be of either sex and there has recently been a strong move by the American Food and Drug Administration to encourage the participation of women in the earliest studies with new drugs. This is a controversial subject and it would be inappropriate to discuss it in detail here but suffice it to say that there is an interval after conception when pregnancy tests are negative and if women capable of child-bearing are to be included there is always a risk of foetal exposure to the drug. The medicolegal implications of this risk generally make pharmaceutical companies and investigators insist that reproductive toxicology studies in particular teratology should be completed before exposure of women.

It is often stated that a healthy or non-patient volunteer cannot be expected to derive any therapeutic benefit from participation in the study. This is true but the corollary which is implied, that patients are likely to derive benefit, is usually incorrect. Whilst a patient in the terminal stages of a fatal disease may have little to lose from trying a new investigational drug and just might stand to gain something, most early drug testing is not intended to demonstrate efficacy and the patients are unlikely to gain directly from partipation in the study. Of course it is possible that if it is successful the patient may eventually be treated with that drug but that is often a remote possibility. All subjects participating in clinical trials are volunteers (or should be) but the distinction between a healthy (non-patient) volunteer and patient volunteer is far from clear when applied to early drug studies.

The choice of the most appropriate study population should be based on ethical, scientific and practical considerations. Clearly there are drugs which should never be given to healthy volunteers such as cytotoxic agents, neuromuscular blocking agents or anaesthetics (in clinically effective doses). Biological response modifiers such as monoclonal antibodies, growth factors and interleukins have been given to healthy subjects but this is controversial. Many antiviral drugs have been studied extensively in healthy volunteers though, for reasons that are not always entirely rational, the first studies of potential treatments for AIDS have usually been conducted in HIV positive individuals. If the availability of patients is not a problem and there is little chance of them being put at significantly greater risk of adverse events because of their disease, it is perfectly reasonable to conduct such studies in the patient population. However, in general, there are a number of advantages of using healthy volunteers as subjects in the first studies of a new active substance which are as follows:

- Recruitment is usually faster than with patients
- Healthy volunteers are usually able to make themselves available on scheduled study days so that groups of subjects can be studied together
- Results are not confounded by effects of the disease, concomitant medications, age and other variables
- Healthy subjects are less likely to suffer consequences of some adverse reactions
- Patients are often less able to cooperate with numerous, complex procedures which these studies may involve

An additional consideration in the UK, though usually more important to a pharmaceutical company than the investigator, is that a clinical trials exemption or certificate (CTX or CTC) is required for most studies in patients but not for healthy volunteers. This may change in the coming years by the implementation of a European Directive for Clinical Trials, which would impose legal requirements on

Box 4.2 Check for minimising risk

- Are the healthy volunteers truly fit to participate in the study?
- Have you made adequate arrangements for medical supervision throughout?
- Are staffing levels adequate and are all staff adequately briefed?
- Are there adequate procedures for checking drug administration?
- Based on preclinical and clinical data, are the selection of starting dose and proposed increments reasonable?
- Is the frequency of vital sign measurements, adverse events probe and other safety measurements adequate?
- Have you taken all the necessary steps to deal with an adverse event and prevent others?
- Have you taken steps to implement interim reviews of data?
- What about medical examinations and blood tests in the follow up period?

all EU countries. The new situation cannot be fully predicted but it will pay to follow developments on the EMEA website (see Chapter 3 for details). Other aspects relating to the recruitment of volunteers are discussed in Chapter 10

The protocol and ethics review

In many respects the protocol for the first administration of a new active substance to man is similar to those of other clinical studies (see Chapter 6) but there are a few important differences and the emphasis is somewhat different. The Ethics Committee bears considerable responsibility in such cases and the protocol should facilitate their decision making. A sponsoring pharmaceutical company should provide an Investigator's Brochure which summarises all the preclinical and clinical information on the drug to date. This does not mean that the protocol need only provide a sketchy outline of important information. While the Investigator's Brochure should be available to the Ethics Committee too, the protocol should be a stand alone document in which there is a comprehensive summary of the most relevant information and any problem areas are highlighted for attention. Description of data should be accompanied by some comments which aid interpretation.

The Committee will need to deliberate on your choice of starting dose and proposed increments so these should be justified. The number of subjects and amount of data that will form the basis for a decision to dose-escalate should be clearly stated and end points for stopping the dose escalation must be clearly defined. These will inevitably include the occurrence of adverse events in one or more subjects which are deemed unacceptable or at least dose-limiting. They may also include attainment of certain values for a pharmacodynamic endpoint or the attainment of a certain plasma concentration of drug or metabolite.

In order to cope with all the unknowns, some degree of flexibility is needed in the protocol so that dose increments and frequency and possibly procedures can be altered or added in the light of new data (See section on Interim Data Review). However, a protocol must define precisely how such interim decisions will be reached and the Ethics Committee may wish to review data as it becomes available and participate in the decision making process.

Interim data review

The principle which must govern all studies in humans but particularly healthy volunteers is that of 'minimal risk'. It is patently obvious that risk can never be reduced to zero when a novel drug is being administered and clinical procedures are being carried out but with due care and attention, risk can truly become minimal. It should be recognised that an ethical study is not necessarily a safe one. Many factors that contribute to safety such as adequate planning, competence of staff, study design and conduct have been discussed in other chapters in this book and are listed in Box 4.2. One which merits some attention here is that of the interim review of data during the course of a study as it is particularly relevant to first administrations.

The latest data should be reviewed after each study day or certainly after a number of volunteers have received a particular dose (the minimum number before dose-escalation should be stated in the protocol). The review should not be a casual affair held between the investigator and a colleague chatting in the corridor but should be a scheduled meeting at which the investigator, study physicians, study nurses and preferably one or two other experienced physicians who are not intimately involved with the study should be present. The Chairman of the Ethics Committee should be informed of the meeting and invited to attend or at least have sight of the data if s/he so wishes. The review requires that all data are collated for presentation which is a useful discipline. Tables and graphs if appropriate should be prepared in advance of the meeting so that there is a real opportunity to scrutinise the data. An agenda should be prepared and notes of decisions taken and action points arising recorded. This documentation is perhaps the most important record of how the study was actually conducted and should be archived in the study file with the case report forms. The agenda for a data review should cover the following:

- Overall progress: number of subject-occasions and doses completed to date
- Adverse events: type, severity, duration, action taken, attributability to drug
- Vital signs and other safety parameters
- Pharmacodynamic measures including biochemical, hormone or other tests of specific relevance to the drug's activity
- Plasma concentrations and pharmacokinetics including issues relating to assay methodology
- Laboratory data: haematology, clinical chemistry, urinalysis etc
- Procedures and methodology

The requirement to have plasma concentrations and pharmacokinetics will perhaps surprise some readers. It certainly places a strain on the bioanalysts but with proper planning and good communication, it should be possible to have rapid (within a few days) turnaround of drug concentration data. Knowledge of maximum concentrations, dose proportionality of area under plasma concentration vs time profiles and half-lives greatly adds to making rational decisions about adverse events and the appropriate next dose-increment. The information can also be used to optimise times for sampling and pharmacodynamic measurements and the appropriate intervals to be allowed between study days and for follow up.

The last item on this list provides an opportunity to review the practical aspects of running the study. This is the opportunity for anyone to speak up with their ideas about how the study can be managed more smoothly.

Research nurses will often have observed that a particular procedure did not go well because insufficient time was allowed or that volunteers were unhappy about the attitude of one of the staff. Laboratory technicians may point out that samples are not being handled in a proficient manner or that the time stagger between subjects is too short to permit processing of the samples.

Not only the quantity and quality of the data may be improved by implementing changes in procedure but also the safety of the volunteers. Any significant modifications to the protocol will need to be submitted to the Ethics Committee and approval obtained before proceeding. The volunteers may also need to be updated about any changes to the schedule and adverse events as the study progresses. As always, a volunteer must be free to withdraw from a study at any stage without prejudice.

Drawing conclusions

Even if a study has achieved all its objectives, the limitations of the first study in man should be recognised. A drug may have been tolerated well by healthy volunteers in the dose-range examined but numbers are small and adverse effects that are not directly related to the drug's pharmacological activity are unlikely to occur. Pharmacokinetic data are of a preliminary nature with perhaps a higher limit of assay quantitation than is ideal and with a less than optimal sampling schedule. Likewise, pharmacodynamic data cannot be definitive without placebo controls. Nevertheless, the information should be of good quality and sufficient for basing a decision on whether to proceed with more definitive studies or whether to stop development of the drug forthwith. Some common reasons for halting drug development at such an early stage are listed in Box 4.3.

If, on the other hand the drug has fulfilled its desired profile, the information will be used to optimise the design of further single and multiple dose studies of tolerability, pharmacokinetics and pharmacodynamic activity and clinical trials of efficacy and safety in the target population.

Box 4.3 Some common reasons for stopping drug development early

- Poorly tolerated in doses/concentrations which are below those expected to be in the therapeutic range
- Inadequate bioavailability to achieve desired plasma concentrations
- Clearance is saturable leading to steep rise of plasma concentrations with small dose increments resulting in adverse effects
- Half life too short so that dosing frequency would be unacceptable
- Multiple metabolites not covered by toxicity studies
- Active metabolites with half lives much longer than parent drug
- Pharmacodynamic activity which forms basis for efficacy is not as expected from animal studies
- Evidence of major organ toxicity eg hepatotoxicity, nephrotoxicity

5

Planning and coordinating the study

Adam Cohen

Introduction

The number of people involved in a clinical study tends to increase as the study progresses from development and ethical clearance of the protocol through the clinical phase, to analysis of results and reporting. This complexity necessitates organisation and management by the investigator.

A clinical study requires careful planning from the moment the initial idea is conceived until the final report has been written. The schedule for the clinical phase of the study should appear in the protocol but that represents only one part of the process. Clear plans are required to organise all the individuals involved and ensure that they are understand fully what is expected of them. Usually, several weeks elapse between submitting the protocol to the ethics committee and receiving approval. This time can be used for detailed planning of the subsequent phases of the study. To avoid errors which may affect the quality of the study data or even put subjects at unnecessary risk one needs to think ahead, spot potential problems and take avoiding action.

Overall study plan

Start by setting a number of milestones which will indicate to you whether things are slipping.

- Deadline for submission of the final protocol
- Date of ethics committee approval
- Proposed start and end dates of clinical phase
- Proposed start and end dates of drug assays
- Proposed start and end dates of pharmacokinetic analysis (if appropriate)
- Proposed start and end dates for statistical analysis
- Deadline for final report

Having set the overall planned dates, practical difficulties will immediately become apparent. For example, the Christmas or summer holidays may be imminent; trials tend not to do well over these periods. Non-permanent staff may be leaving before the end of the study or may have other work commitments. It is useful to make lists of these points.

Checklists and planning charts are useful tools to track progress. An examples of a checklist for a clinical study is shown in Box 5.1. Obviously they can be modified to fit your own particular requirements. The checklist is simple but may rapidly be covered with crossings out and rewritten dates so that before too long it becomes unintelligible. Gant planning charts can be drawn by hand but various software packages are available for project planning and production of clear planning charts. Clearly, access to a computer and some investment of money, time and effort are required but the great advantage is that the knock on effect of one date slipping on all subsequent activities is easily demonstrated and, unlike humans, the computer will not make errors in its calculations (Figure 5.1). However a simple list will do as well in many cases-provided you use it and take action when things do not go the way you expected.

Staff It is unreasonable to expect colleagues, commonly junior staff, who have other full time work commitments to help you conduct a clinical study without adequate prior warning. A careful breakdown of the study is required. Don't underestimate the work-load which tends to increase as the study progresses.

- Assess the number and type of personnel required to run the study. Staff that will be required are likely to belong to one of the following groups:
  - Clinical: physicians, nurses, technicians
  - Administrative: secretaries, data typists
  - Pharmaceutical company: physicians, monitor
  - Laboratory: scientists, technicians
  - Pharmacists
- Having decided on the appropriate composition of the team before the study starts provide them with information. You may have been involved in the details of the study for a long time, but the others staff may not know much about it. Nurses often play an essential role in a clinical study but they tend to receive inadequate information. It is useful to have at least two meetings

before the study, one in which you give general information to a larger group and one *pre start* meeting during which you assess if all details are in place. This takes place approximately one week before patient recruitment starts. During the study you have to keep everyone informed at regular intervals.

Box 5.1 Project administration

Project number:	Date registered:	
Title:		
Project leader:		
Sponsor:		
Collaborating departments:		
	Plan	Actual
Registration		
Study summary		
Final protocol		
Internal review		
Approved internally		
To ethics committee		
Approval ethics committee		
Start clinical phase		
End clinical phase		
Data analysis		
Date final report		
Submission of publication		
Acceptance by journal		
Archiving of study data		

Figure 5A Gant chart demonstrating a study plan

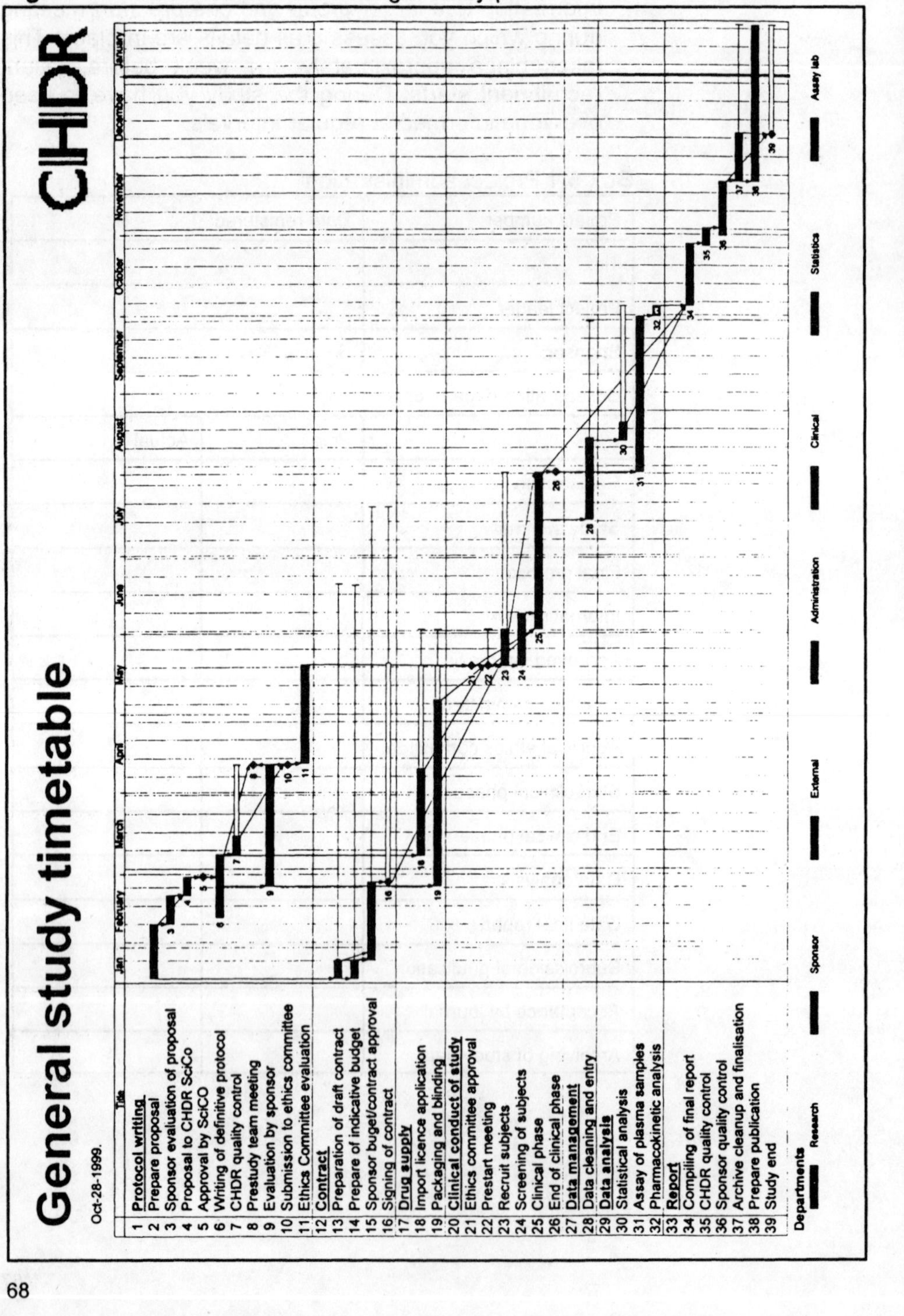

Box 5.2 Study budget

item	number	cost/item	TOTAL
Personnel - medical			
Personnel - nursing			
Personnel - administrative			
Other personnel costs (travel etc)			
Accommodation - hospital bed days			
Drugs - purchase and preparation			
Laboratory costs (reagent kits)			
Assays - clinical chemistry/hematology			
Disposables (syringes, sample tubes)			
Travel costs subjects			
Stationery - (printed trial material)			
Capital equipment (or depreciation)			
TOTAL FUNDING REQUIRED			

Laboratory support

Make sure you inform the laboratory about all work in which they are involved. This includes routine haematology and clinical chemistry. It is easy to underestimate the amount of time involved in laboratory analysis of the sizable number of samples that can be generated during trials. It is not a good idea to turn up at the laboratory with a large batch of samples without prior warning.

- How should samples be handled? What anticoagulant is required for blood samples? Do containers for urine collections need to contain an antioxidant or other preservative? Do blood samples need to be separated immediately in a refrigerated centrifuge or can they stand at room temperature and be centrifuged some time later?
- Samples will have to be stored during the study and

often for a long time afterwards. Freezer space is limited, and an assessment of the total number of samples and their storage conditions can be used to estimate requirements. It may be necessary to obtain a freezer that is dedicated to the study. This may have implications for your budget and can be estimated long before the need arises!

- How long will it take to complete the analyses? This will obviously depend on the number of samples as well as the complexity of any extraction procedure and type of assay. Do the samples have to be analysed rapidly or can they be stored until the end of the study and then batch processed? What is the capacity of the laboratory with regard to staff and equipment?
- Having established the planned duration of storage, it is essential to verify that the samples are stable for such a period.

Drug supply and packing This is often forgotten until the last moment. It is essential to consider the following points well before the trial is about to start.

- Do not consider dispensing drug yourself; ask a pharmacist to help. Preparation of drugs requires great precision and tends to be a source of errors when performed by other personnel.
- Is the amount of drug available and sufficient for the planned number of trial subjects?
- Is the drug stable for the expected period of the study (and for longer, since most studies take longer than expected). Are there special storage conditions and can you comply with them?
- What is the situation with regard to importing the drug if it has to come from abroad?
- The drugs should be packed in individual packs for each patient that are designed to ensure compliance with the prescribed dosage schedule. When complicated regimes are used special calendar or blister packs may be required; these take time to prepare. Packing for double blind studies can be very complicated and early contact with the pharmacist is mandatory.
- Intravenous injections may have to be prepared shortly before administration and some drugs (cytostatics)

have to be prepared in special conditions.

Source of subjects and expected recruitment rate

Healthy volunteers are generally more readily available than patients. Most people overestimate the number of patients that can be recruited. Probably more trials fail through over optimistic predictions about patient number than anything else; patient recruitment should therefore be monitored closely. An initial assessment of recruitment should have been made when writing the protocol, but this should be reevaluated.

- The protocol should give the total number of subjects to be recruited.
- Plan your weekly or monthly recruitment rate.
- Compare predicted with actual numbers frequently. This requires courage and may be disappointing! For larger studies a graph may be useful.
- Take action if things are going too slowly.

Funding

It is important to ensure funding for the study and every study should have a budget. The following (by no means exhaustive) list (Box 5.2) gives a number of points to take into account when determining the cost of a study. Make a budget for each year (or other period), to find out when costs are incurred you can use the planning charts.

Administrative planning

Every clinical study tends to generate a surprising amount of paper. The unprepared investigator is easily swamped by this. As the study progresses no time can be found to put this in order. This requires preparation before the study starts.

Keep all correspondence and other documents related to the study in a ringbinder - the *trial file*. When a department runs more than one study at a time, it is useful to devise a system of study numbers and keep the different trial files together (for example in the secretariat). Do not keep results in these folders. Data should be kept in a more secure place. The trial file can be subdivided into the following sections:

- General study planning (see above)
- Contact addresses and telephone numbers
- Correspondence in/out
- Protocol (as approved by the ethics committee)

- Protocol amendments
- Data collection forms
- Randomisation list (in the case of a double blind only to be added at the end of the study)
- Emergency code for double blind studies
- Budget and finance
- Contracts with sponsoring drug company or funding charity
- Patient information sheet and informed consent
- Drug quality control certificates
- Monitoring reports
- Curriculum vitae of investigators
- List of members of ethics committee
- Final report and publications

The file can be archived when the study is complete. Such a file ensures that up-to-date administrative information is available to everyone concerned. As the review process of the study progresses numerous small changes in the protocol may be necessary. It is essential to keep track of these in the trial file and to make sure that the last version of the protocol is always available.

Overall checklist

- Overall study plan
- Budget and funding arranged
- Subject recruitment
- Staff and team composition
- Pre start meeting arranged
- Laboratory support arranged
- Drug import licence
- Drug supply and packing
- Administrative
- Data collection

Finally, everyone is interested in the results of the study. This includes the patients who will appreciate a short letter with a summary of the results.

6

The study protocol

John Posner and Ria Kroon

What is a protocol?

The essential elements of a protocol are:

- A scientific rationale
- The objectives of the proposed study
- A description of the study population
  - Inclusion and exclusion criteria for recruitment of subjects
  - The number of subjects to be recruited
- A precise description of the procedures that will be performed including:
  - Dosages of drugs that will be administered
  - Volumes of blood to be sampled
  - What will be assayed in these samples
  - Measurements that will be made to assess drug effects
  - The times at which all procedures will be done
  - How long and under what conditions subjects will be studied

Protocols emanating from pharmaceutical companies often run to 50 pages or more. Whilst independent academic investigators sometimes feel that the industry is excessively bureaucratic when it comes to documentation, it should be appreciated that there are real advantages to writing a good protocol. Attention to detail at this early stage will maximise the chances of the study actually providing the answers to the questions that it is intended to address. Sloppiness in the protocol is likely to translate into unnecessary variability of data and failure to provide meaningful results and could result in participating subjects being put at unnecessary risk.

It must also be recognised that a protocol for a study to be conducted in humans is a legal document with regulatory and medico-legal implications. As with any legal document ambiguity and vagueness are to be avoided.

Who reads the protocol?

There are many interested parties who need to read this document. The ethics and safety considerations are the particular concern of the Ethics Committee whose primary role is to safeguard patients and healthy volunteers participating in the study. Clinical research nurses and technicians must be able to follow the schedule and be fully familiar with the methodology so that every procedure can be performed as described in the protocol. This also applies to laboratory scientists responsible for carrying out drug assays, biochemical, haematological, immunological or other tests. A pharmaceutical company monitor (see Chapter 11) will need to be fully familiar with the protocol in order to ensure that the investigator is complying with the protocol and that the Case Report Forms are being completed correctly. Drug regulatory authorities and those responsible for making submissions to these authorities on behalf of pharmaceutical companies or contract research organisations will be particularly concerned about compliance, ie. is what is written in the protocol what was actually done and if not, how significant were the protocol deviations? Finally, because the investigator is often not the author of the protocol, it is necessary to state that the investigator himself needs to be fully conversant with the details of the protocol. He or she must know precisely what is involved, that the study is practicable given the availability of subjects, facilities, equipment, staff and time and that the study is ethical.

Who writes the protocol?

To some extent, the authorship of the protocol depends on circumstances. If an academic clinical scientist wishes to carry out a piece of experimental work in humans on their own initiative, that individual will be responsible for writing the protocol. Alternatively, when a study is to be carried out on behalf of a pharmaceutical company for drug regulatory purposes, it is common for personnel in the company to write the protocol and then to agree it with the investigator. Frequently, pharmaceutical companies carry out multi-centre studies with many investigators. It is essential for the company that a single protocol is used and they will understandably be reluctant to change a protocol to satisfy a particular investigator when the same protocol has been found acceptable to other investigators. Sometimes the clinical phase of the study may have already started in other centres but good companies will confer with their potential investigators and obtain expert opinion well in advance so that the design of the study can be optimised and major problems arising at a late stage can be avoided. Of course no investigator should agree to a protocol which is significantly flawed with respect to scientific justification or study design or is simply impracticable.

There are a variety of ways of writing a protocol and the precise order of the various sections and how they are grouped is a matter of individual taste. Many pharmaceutical companies standardise the format of their documents. An example of a tried and tested format is given below. Whatever arrangement is preferred, almost all the sections listed are essential. The ICH-GCP guidelines also give a suggested set of headings for a study protocol.

Title page

This should give:

- Title of the protocol
- The date of the current version of the protocol
- Names and qualifications of authors
- Name and qualifications of principal and other investigators,
- Name, address and phone number of institution where the study will be conducted
- The name, title, address and phone number of the person responsible for the medical care of the subjects (if someone other than the investigator)
- The names and addresses of the laboratories and/or other technical departments involved in the execution of the protocol

If the study is being sponsored by a pharmaceutical company, the title page should also give:

- The name and address of the sponsor
- Names and titles of the persons authorised to sign the protocol and amendments on behalf of the sponsor.
- The name of the trial monitor(s)
- The name, title and phone number of the medical expert of the sponsor to be contacted in case of serious adverse events

The protocol will also be given a number for the company's documentation records management. When the study is conducted by the investigator without a sponsor it is also advisable to develop a system of protocol numbers for internal use.

Summary
This should be no more than a page or two giving the essential features of the study. It can be set out as a series of brief statements headed as follows:

- Rationale
- Objectives
- Design
- Setting
- Study population
- Measurements
- Data analysis

It may also be appropriate to mention any specific major considerations about drug dosages and safety.

Contents
Self-explanatory.

List of abbreviations
Don't assume that the local jargon is familiar to all readers and list all the abbreviations that are used in the protocol, except commonly used SI (Système Internationale) units.

1. Introduction and rationale
This is the scientific background and justification for the study. Its length will depend on the complexity of the study and how much background information is really new rather than common knowledge. It may suffice to give a fairly brief scientific rationale and justification for a study which uses standard clinical procedures and marketed pharmaceutical medicines. By contrast, a study of a new molecular entity will require a considerable amount of background information relating to pharmacology and toxicology in animals as well as experience in humans. However, for even the simplest study, the scientific rationale, which constitutes the justification for performing the study, should be well argued with adequate referencing of the published literature.

2. Objectives
A brief statement of one, two or three precise objectives of

the study (see Chapter 7). There is no place for a long wish list or ambiguity here as the final conclusions of the study when reported should relate back directly to the objectives.

3. Study design

One or two paragraphs defining exactly the design of the study:

- The study population whether healthy volunteers or patients, whether it is to be cross-over or parallel groups
- Randomised or not
- Open, single-blind or double-blind
- Placebo and/or positive control or comparator treatment
- Duration and number of study occasions
- A list of drugs and placebo that will be administered and dosages
- Tests that will be performed and measurements made

It is good practice to add a paragraph or two to this section relating to particular design considerations such as the reason for selecting particular drug dosage, pharmaceutical formulation, dosage intervals and period of drug administration, particular safety considerations and, most importantly, a statement about the statistical power which justifies the size of population to be studied. The absence of a power calculation may mean that the study has no chance of showing differences which comprise the objectives of the study because the number of subjects is too small. Such a study is not only a waste of effort but also unethical. Conversely, it is just as wrong to expose an unnecessarily large number of subjects to a new drug or potentially hazardous procedure.

4. Subjects, screening, consent and clearance procedures

4.1 Subjects. Their number and demographic features such as age, sex, range of acceptable body weights, smokers or not and whether healthy or patients with a particular disease. The source of subjects should also be given eg. a panel of healthy volunteers, patients from a particular clinic etc. Details of the recruitment procedures should be provided and, if a notice is to be used to advertise the study, this must be referred to and included as an appendix to the protocol.

4.2 Inclusion and exclusion criteria. This section will define precisely who is eligible to enter the study. Healthy volunteers should be just that and there is little room for flexibility; the criteria should be very strict. With regard to patient populations, it may be desirable to cast the net as wide as possible but failure to recruit a defined population may well render the study useless. On the other hand, criteria which are too strict may make it impossible to recruit at a reasonable speed and may result in the population not being representative of the patient population of interest. Exclusion criteria will usually include pregnancy, certain diseases and known allergy to drugs belonging to the class that is being studied. Lack of eligibility also arises from unwillingness of the volunteer to comply with the terms of the study which may involve restrictions such as abstaining from coffee or alcohol or the requirement to attend for follow up on certain days. Concomitant medications which are permitted and others that are specifically excluded should be listed. There may also be a need for specific exclusions amongst the potential study population such as patients who have the disease but in a form which is insufficiently severe to permit benefit to be measured or conversely whose prognosis is so bad that the therapeutic intervention would not receive a fair test or would be un-ethical. A useful rule is to nominate as entry criteria those that will allow you to make the initial selection from the general population. Normally the subjects can themselves determine whether they satisfy the entry criteria. Exclusion criteria are applied to this group and are generally determined by the physician. Using these definitions age, sex, smoking status are entry criteria, but blood pressure, plasma creatinine etc are exclusion criteria.

4.3 Screening. The procedure should be described precisely with a list of investigations that will be performed. A typical list for healthy volunteers and many patients is as follows:

- Medical history
- Physical examination
- Electrocardiogram
- Full blood count

- Plasma biochemistry profile (detailed list)
- Plasma virological tests for evidence of Hepatitis B and C and HIV infection.
- Urine drug screen (detailed list)
- Urinalysis
- Pregnancy test

Additional tests for certain studies might include Holter monitor for 24 hour cardiac arrhythmia analysis, spirometry, coagulation tests, creatinine clearance and of course specific tests for diagnosis or assessment of the severity of a disease.

4.4 Informed consent (see Chapter 9). Procedures for obtaining consent should include a description of how the subject will learn of the study eg advertisement, notice posted on board in clinic and how they will receive detailed information about it. Written information must be made available with or as part of the consent form and this, together with any notice should appear as appendices to the protocol (see below). It should be stated that the opportunity for subjects to ask questions and receive clear answers from the investigator will be provided. The actual time when written consent will be requested and who will witness this, should be identified.

4.5 Withdrawal of subjects. It should be stated clearly that subjects have the right to withdraw at any time without prejudice and without giving a reason. The responsible physician also has the right to withdraw a subject; the reasons for such a withdrawal should be recorded.

4.6 Honorarium. It should be stated whether an honorarium is to be paid to healthy volunteers and, if so, how much. This also applies to small gifts or tokens. It is not usual to pay an honorarium to patients but they may receive expenses including loss of earnings; this also should be stated clearly. Increasingly, ethics committees are interested in the honorarium paid to the investigator as well.

4.7 Compensation for injury. If your arrangements comply with the guidelines on the terms and conditions for compensation for injury incurred in clinical trials, make a clear statement about this here.

4.8 Clearance procedures. The individuals or bodies required to review and approve the protocol should be identified. This not only includes the name of the Ethics Committee or Institutional Review Board but also may involve internal approval procedures within a pharmaceutical company or academic institution. If a new molecular entity (unlicensed) is to be tested in patients, it will generally be necessary to clear the protocol with a regulatory authority and in some countries (the USA among others) this also applies to healthy volunteers. In the UK protocols for studies involving administration of radioactive materials need to be submitted to the Administration of Radioactive Substances Committee (ARSAC) together with the calculations for exposure.

5. Formulations, drugs and dosages

Details should be provided of the manufacturer and supply of drug and related materials, how they will be packed and presented eg coded vials or containers with individual subject numbers, study days, storage conditions and how they will be accounted for. Sometimes it is appropriate to give precise details of the drug and excipients contained in the formulation. There should always be a precise description of the conditions under which drug will be administered, e.g. capsule to be swallowed with 200 ml water after an overnight fast in the presence of physician or nurse, infusion of concentration 1 mg/ml at 2 ml/h for 3 hours, 2 tablets to be self administered every 12 hours with meals for 5 days for a total of 10 doses (20 tablets). Occasionally, a physician or pharmacist has to be unblinded in order to prepare a weight adjusted dose of diluted drug for parenteral administration. In this case, the individual should be identified in the protocol and the measures that will be taken to avoid bias and unblinding of other personnel should be specified.

6. Measurements and evaluations

6.1 Schedule. A detailed listing of the days, hours and minutes when clinical procedures will be carried out. The time of every blood sample, blood pressure measurement and examination should be given such that nurses, technicians, physicians and other staff can follow it precisely. Remember it takes a finite amount of time to measure a blood pressure or to provide a urine specimen and nothing can be done at the same time. If several subjects are to be studied on a single day with times staggered, the exact times for each subject should be charted so that overlaps and potential clashes where staff or subjects would need to be in two places at once can be avoided. Restrictions on subjects such as fasting overnight before study days, abstaining from caffeine-containing products, alcohol etc and precautions like not driving or operating machinery need to be detailed here as well as in the written information that will be provided to the subjects. It is good practice to give the schedule to the subjects with the other written information as well as to staff so that they know exactly what is involved.The expected duration of subject participation and the sequence and duration of all trial periods, including, if appropriate, follow-up, should also be described.

6.2 Clinical procedures. The purpose of this section is to delineate methodology that will be employed in the Study Unit or Clinic. Every procedure should be described including cannulation, blood sampling, electrocardiograms, blood pressures, urine collections, lung function tests etc. It is not good enough simply to state that blood pressure will be measured or heart rate recorded. Blood pressure may be measured at different sites (brachial, finger etc) using a variety of apparatus (random zero sphygmomanometer, automated oscillometric devices etc). Heart rate may be counted at the radial pulse for a variable period of time, determined from the average of 10 consecutive beats of the electrocardiogram and so on. Any rating scales used for evaluation should be explained. If subjects will be self-administering medication, methods to check compliance should be described.

6.3 Laboratory procedures. This has the same purpose as the previous section and relates to assays of drugs and metabolites, haematology, clinical biochemistry investigations etc.

6.4 Adverse experiences. A description of how data on adverse experiences will be acquired eg spontaneous reporting, check lists administered at specified times, etc and procedures for recording and handling them. The period of recording adverse experiences is worth documenting to avoid arbitrary decisions having to be made about this. In many drug studies, it is reasonable to use the same period as that of blood sampling. Procedures to be followed in the event of a serious adverse experience (life-threatening or significantly disabling or requiring hospitalisation) should be stated.

6.5 Comedication and other treaments

A description of permitted and not permitted comedication and other treatments (before the start and during the execution of the study) should be included in the protocol.

6.6 Procedures for monitoring subject compliance

When the trial is analysed it is of the utmost importance to know if the treatments were actually taken by the subjects. This is particularly relevant when part or all of the trial takes place on an out-patient basis. The methodology employed to check on compliance (e.g. tablet counts, plasma concentration monitoring, electronic devices etc) should be stated.

7. Data management and analysis

It is important to describe how data from different sources will be entered into a data base, spreadsheet or whatever and whether such systems have been validated. Data collected on case report forms may have to be entered manually while data acquired by computer or dedicated electronic devices and from laboratories may be downloaded directly. It is not adequate to state that results will be analysed by standard statistical methods. The comparisons that will be made, the selection of subjects to be included in the analysis (eg all subjects receiving investigational drug, all subjects that received a randomisation code, etc), the statistical techniques that are likely to be used in the analysis and, if appropriate, the timepoints of interim analysis should be described after consultation with a statistician who will be involved in the analysis.

For pharmacokinetics, the programs that will be used

for analysis should be identified, whether non-compartmental or model-dependent methods will be employed, how parameters will be calculated, whether they will be log transformed and what comparisons will be made.

8. Study management

8.1 Records management. How subject numbering and identification will be maintained and source document verification carried out. There should also be a description of how records will be stored during and after the trial, how confidentiality will be maintained and who will have access to the records.

8.2 Randomisation code. Who will generate the code, who will keep copies (sealed), safeguards for maintaining the blind and procedures for accessing and breaking the code in the event of an emergency.

8.3 Patient withdrawal or discontinuation of the study. Procedures to be followed and criteria for withdrawal of subjects and criteria for premature discontinuation of the study may need to be specified.

8.4 Study personnel and responsibilities. This will include the names of the trial monitor if appropriate and physician responsible for the welfare of subjects with details of how long the physician will be present in the Clinic or Study Unit after dosing and how he can be contacted at other times.

8.5 Audit. A brief statement that the trial may be audited by an external body such as a regulatory authority or, if appropriate audited by a sponsor's quality assurance department and that the raw data will also be inspected.

9. QA and QC procedures

A description of the QA and QC procedures to be performed at the investigational site.

10. Publication Policy

Especially when partners from different organisations participate in a study, interests in publishing the data may vary considerably. This needs to be clearly laid down before the results are available and does not only apply to industry-academia partnerships.

11. References

This is a listing of all referenced work in the protocol using Vancouver Format (see Chapter 12).

12. Tables

13. Figures

14. Appendices

The appendices required will naturally depend on circumstances but should generally include:

- The notice or advertisement that will be displayed to attract potential volunteers
- The written information that will be provided to potential volunteers with the consent form
- The letter that will be sent to the volunteer's general practitioner

Other appendices may include special diet sheets, rating scales, details of assay procedures, mathematical equations for calculation of results to be derived from data acquired etc.

Protocol amendments

After a protocol has been submitted and cleared by an Ethics Committee or Regulatory Authority, it is not a simple matter to amend it. Any amendments need to be approved by the body in question and this can take time and may delay the start of a study significantly. Prevention is better than cure so that when it is foreseeable that a procedure may change during the course of a study it is better to state this in the original protocol. Whilst an Ethics Committee should not be giving carte blanche to an investigator, it is perfectly reasonable that permission be given in advance to change some sampling times after obtaining preliminary assay data providing this will not lead to additional blood loss or for the interval between study days to be lengthened because the half-life of a drug is longer than expected. In other situations it may be totally inappropriate for there to be any flexibility in a protocol and any changes will need to be submitted as formal protocol amendments so it is worth trying hard to get it right first time. Having dealt with the formal side of an amendment does not mean your work is over. You will also have to communicate the change to all involved in the trial and ensure that all participants work with the same version of the protocol

7

Study Design

Les Huson

Introduction

Clinical studies are undertaken in order to reach some conclusion about a treatment regime, and it is generally intended that this conclusion should be widely applicable - at least, to a larger group of patients than that studied in the trial itself. The patients recruited into the study therefore constitute just a sample of all of the patients to whom the investigational treatment regime might eventually be applied. This raises two questions: firstly, how can this sample be selected so that it is in some sense representative of the larger group of patients, and secondly, how can the data from the sample be analysed in a way which will yield conclusions that might validly be applied to the larger group of patients?

The answers to these two questions are the province of clinical statistics; the principles and methods of statistical design attempt to answer the first question, and the principles and methods of statistical analysis attempt to answer the second. This chapter is concerned with principles of statistical design; statistical analysis is discussed in Chapter 8.

Good statistical design is largely a matter of logic and organisation - most good clinical studies are simple and straightforward in their construction and execution - and it helps to have a logical sequence of steps when designing a study. The checklist in Box 7.1 shows such a logical sequence. The steps in this sequence are discussed in more detail below.

Objectives

Every well-designed clinical study should have clear objectives. If no objectives are specified, it will be impossible to be sure that an efficient study design has been selected, and it will be impossible for others to judge, after the trial has completed, whether or not it was conducted efficiently. A trial is only good to the extent that it meets its objectives, though serendipity may occasionally result in a trial producing an interesting and

Box 7.1 Logical sequence in clinical study

- Define and write down a clear set of objectives
- Define the patient population
- Choose control treatments with which the experimental therapy is to be compared
- Choose an appropriate trial structure
- Select an appropriate sample size
- Organise the blinding and randomisation procedures

useful result despite poor design.

Objectives should be clear and specific, and they should be written down in the study protocol. They should refer to definite measurements and endpoints. For example, in a trial studying hypertension, a good objective might use the phrase '... to compare the reductions in systolic blood pressure over a 6 month period achieved by treatment A and treatment B'. A poor and vague objective, sadly often encountered, might simply say '.... to compare the efficacy of treatment A and treatment B'.

Ideally, a trial should not have too many objectives. If it does, it generally becomes difficult to optimise the design, since attempting to achieve several different objectives will often place too many constraints on the way the trial is structured. If there are several objectives, it is helpful to specify them in order of priority.

Specification of clear objectives does not prohibit additional exploration of the data once the study has finished. In fact, such exploration is generally a good idea, since every opportunity should be taken to extract as much information from a study as possible. However, exploratory analyses - analyses done in addition to those which are designed to meet the specified objectives - have a different statistical interpretation, and must therefore be clearly identified as such.

Defining the patient population

When the trial is concluded, it is hoped that certain conclusions can be reached about the effectiveness of the study drug. To which patients can these conclusions validly be applied? The obvious answer is that the conclusions apply to all patients 'similar' to those included in the study, but unless there is a clear definition of the criteria by which patients were selected, it will remain unclear who these 'similar' patients are. Patient selection is best organised by drawing up a list of inclusion and exclusion criteria; these are not just there to assist the investigator in screening patients - they have a clear statistical interpretation in that they *define* the patient population that is being studied.

The nature of these criteria will naturally vary from study to study, depending on the nature of the disease and the drug under investigation. Generally, though, the criteria will involve such things as ages of patients, disease severity or symptoms or stage of disease progression, and will often restrict the use of alternative or concomitant drug treatments. In early stages of drug development, when less is known of the safety of the drug, it is often the case that women of childbearing potential are excluded from investigational studies.

There is sometimes the temptation, in drawing up a list of inclusion criteria, to restrict the types of patients who are deemed eligible in a way which will maximise the chances of success of the experimental therapy; there is no reason in principle why this should not be done, but it must be remembered that the conclusions reached in the study may only validly be applied to other similar patients - so if a highly restricted group is used in the study, the conclusions apply only to other patients exhibiting a similarly restricted range of characteristics.

Control treatments

With a clear set of objectives, and a definition of the type of patient to be included in the trial, the next step in planning is to select appropriate control treatments with which the experimental therapy may be compared.

There are two types of control treatment: placebo and active. A third possibility, which should ideally be avoided, but which is sometimes unavoidable, is to use no control treatment at all. Placebo controls are appropriate in cases in which there is no generally accepted standard therapy against which the experimental approach can be compared. An active control is usually used if there is a generally accepted standard therapy for the condition being studied, and in such cases the experimental drug will be compared with the active standard either to establish whether or not it is superior, or at least to establish whether or not it can be considered to be equivalent (the objectives of the study should state which of these two conclusions the trial is attempting to reach). Sometimes it will be appropriate to use both a placebo control and an active control in the same study; sometimes more than one active control may be indicated, or more than one dose level of either active control and/or test drug.

Box 7.2 Parallel and cross-over study designs

Parallel design

Patients group 1	Treatment A
Patients group 2	Treatment B
Group 3,4 etc	Treatment C, D
	Time ➤➤➤➤

Cross-over design

Group 1	Treatment A	Treatment B	Treatment C etc
Group 2	Treatment B	Treatment A	Treatment C etc
Group 3, 4	Treatment C	Treatment B	Treatment A etc
		Time ➤➤➤➤	

Trial structure The next stage in planning a study is to select an appropriate trial structure. The literature in clinical trials contains many examples of unusual and occasionally ingenious trial designs, but there are two standards, widely used and with well-understood properties, one of which will be appropriate in almost all cases. In most cases it makes sense to select one of these two standards, so that the results of the trial will be more easily understood and more readily and widely accepted. The more esoteric the design, the more scope there is for sceptical criticism of the results once the trial has finished. The two 'gold standards' are *parallel* trials and *cross-over* trials. A parallel trial involves the use of two or more concurrently studied groups of patients, each group receiving one of the possible treatments being studied. In a cross-over study, there are also two or more groups of patients, but each group receives two or more of the possible treatments administered in a pre-defined sequence, generally with a specified interval of time - a 'washout-period' - separating each of the different treatments. The structures are shown diagrammatically in Box 7.2.

Parallel trials are appropriate in all circumstances in which the disease state is relatively short-term, potentially curable, or potentially lethal. In all these cases, the likelihood is that there may only be an opportunity to administer one treatment to a patient, not a sequence of treatments. In cases where the disease state is chronic, unlikely to change over time, and likely to return to its initial state once treatment is withdrawn, a cross-over study is possible.

Box 7.3 Choosing between a parallel and a cross-over study

Summary of criteria and trial properties

Parallel trial is essential:

- If the disease is short-term, or potentially curable by the treatment, or potentially lethal

Parallel trial is desirable:

- Even if the disease state is chronic
- In cases where long treatment periods are required (e.g. longer than 3 months)
- Where there are more than 3 treatments to be compared

Cross-over trial is possible:

- when the disease state is chronic and will return to its pre-treatment state when a treatment is finished
- for up to 3 treatments (more are possible but not desirable) provided that it can be demonstrated that treatment effects will not carry-over from one treatment period to a subsequent one

Parallel trials are:

- Generally to be preferred
- Likely to require more patients than a cross-over
- Less likely to suffer complications in trial execution
- Less likely to suffer large numbers of patient-withdrawals
- Likely to be shorter
- Likely to be easier to analyse statistically

Cross-over trials are:

- Second choice!
- Likely to require fewer patients
- More likely to be difficult to execute
- More likely to suffer patient withdrawals
- Likely to be longer overall

More likely to be complicated to analyse and interpret

Parallel studies are generally considered to be the

preferred option, especially by national drug-regulatory authorities, and for this reason alone a parallel study should be selected if possible, but one of the main reasons why cross-overs are sometimes preferred is that a parallel study will generally require the use of a larger sample of patients. Cross-over trials are mainly avoided because of the difficulties of showing firstly that the effect of a treatment does not 'carry-over' into the next stage of the trial, when the next drug is administered, and secondly of showing that the disease itself is returning to the 'pre-treatment' state during each washout period. Box 7.3 has a checklist suggesting criteria for choosing between a parallel and a cross-over trial.

Pre-determined sample sizes and other stopping-rules

It is essential that, before a trial is started, rules are specified for determining when the trial will stop. Such rules must be specified in advance, otherwise the results of the study become difficult or impossible to interpret.

The simplest and most widely used 'stopping-rule' is to specify in advance how many patients will be recruited into the study, and to stop when that number has been recruited. Trials conducted in this way are known as 'fixed-sample' studies. The alternative is to specify that the trial will stop when certain results have been achieved; this means looking at the accumulating data during the course of the trial, analysing the data to determine whether this pre-specified result has been achieved or not, and either continuing with the trial or stopping it, depending upon the results of the analysis. Such studies are known as 'sequential' trials. Sometimes these two types of rule are combined, so that the trial will stop *either* if a certain result is achieved at an 'interim-analysis', or, otherwise, after a fixed number of patients have been recruited.

Fixed sample studies are administratively straightforward, and also easier to plan and analyse statistically. It is simply a matter of calculating how many patients to recruit into the study!

Before such a calculation can be made, it is necessary to make an informed guess about the probable outcome of the trial. This may initially seem odd - the argument is often heard that if the probable outcome was known, there would be no need to conduct the trial. However, it is again a matter of logic: if nothing at all can be said about the outcome, how could it be possible to judge whether or not the trial will have enough patients? To determine a sample size in advance, it is usually necessary to estimate the probable response rate on the experimental therapy, the probable response rate on the control therapy, and also, in many cases, to estimate the likely variability of the responses from patient to patient. Given such information, simple formulae and tables can be used to indicate how many patients should be recruited into the trial, in order to give a 'high probability' that the trial will terminate with a statistically significant result. The 'high probability' referred to here is technically known as the 'power' of the study; for example, in a trial of two treatments, one of which is expected to produce a response in 50% of patients, and the other expected to produce a response in 40% of patients, it can be calculated that a trial with a total sample size of 1040 patients (520 in each group) would have 90% power to yield a statistically significant result (the statistical significance being 0.05, two-tailed - see below). A rough and suitable interpretation of this statement for practical purposes is that there is a 90% chance that a trial of such a size would produce a significant result, given that the assumptions made about likely responses were accurate.

Sample size calculations can be performed for a variety of different possible types of outcome e.g. comparisons of mean values of an endpoint, comparison of proportions of successful responses, comparisons of survival times. In each case, some preliminary estimates of likely outcomes will be needed. Detailed tables and formulae for a variety of sample size calculation problems can be found in Machin and Campbell (1993).

In all cases, the sample sizes derived from such calculations should be treated as approximations only; this is partly because the initial estimates of likely outcomes may be unduly optimistic, but also because certain statistical assumptions and approximations are usually made in the formulae and tables used for the calculations. It is a good idea to round up the numbers derived from such calculations, and also, if possible, recruit some additional patients to cover any whose responses cannot be evaluated due, perhaps, to protocol violations or to early withdrawal from the study.

Sequential trials, or trials with interim analyses, need careful statistical construction and professional advice must be used in their design. The main advantage of such trials is that there is a good chance (but *not* a guarantee) that they may reach a definite conclusion with fewer patients than would be necessary for a fixed sample study. The magnitude of this 'good chance' will vary from study to study, and it is possible for a statistician to estimate the probability that such a study would finish earlier than its fixed-sample equivalent. There are a large number of statistical theories, methods and plans for interim analyses and sequential trials; an up-to-date and largely unified approach to this type of trial design is given by Whitehead (1992); this approach to interim and sequential analyses has the advantage that it is supported by a readily available software package to assist in statistical design and analysis (Brunier and Whitehead, 1993).

Randomisation and blinding

The next stage in the design of a study is to determine the randomisation and blinding methods. In a trial with more than one treatment (or treatment sequence in the case of a cross-over study), it is necessary to assign recruited patients *at random* to one of the possible treatments (or treatment sequences). This avoids the bias that would almost inevitably result if investigators were allowed to choose which patient was allocated to which treatment. However, it isn't just a matter of avoiding bias in allocation of patients to treatments - the statistical methods which will be used to analyse the resulting data will be based on mathematical theories which will assume that random allocation has been used. If patients are not randomly assigned to treatment, then such analyses would be invalid.

Random allocation of patients to treatment is done in practice using computer programs which generate a randomisation code; such a code consists, in its simplest form, of a list of patient numbers, and a corresponding list identifying which treatment should be given to a each patient. When a patient is recruited into the study, he/she is assigned the next available patient number, and given the treatment associated with that number.

In most cases, treatments are not identified explicitly on randomisation codes - instead, an arbitrary letter is used, so that a treatment will be identified only as 'Treatment A', for example. Similarly, the packaged drug will often be labelled only with a code of this kind, so that neither the patient nor the investigator knows the actual identity of the treatment that is being administered. This principle is called 'blinding'. In an 'open' or 'unblinded' study, the patient and the investigator both know which treatment the patient is receiving. This is simple to administer, but it is well known that a knowledge of the identity of the administered treatment may influence either the patient's response, or at least influence the patient's or the investigator's assessment of the response. For this reason, unblinded studies should be avoided.

A second possibility is to keep the patient unaware of the identity of the treatment being administered, but allow the investigator to know. Such trials are called 'single-blind'. They may be suitable if the response being measured is very objective, but may still be susceptible to bias because of the investigator's knowledge. Sometimes open or single-blind trials can be made 'blind at randomisation'; this means that the identity of the allocated treatment is coded until such time as a patient number has been assigned, and an associated treatment identified. After it has been determined, for example, that the patient is to receive 'Treatment 1', the code can be unblinded to reveal the true identity of 'Treatment 1' either to patient, to investigator, or to both. For such blind randomisation to be effective, each individual drug pack must have a unique number, and a separate list prepared identifying specific treatments with specific pack numbers.

It is, however, widely accepted that the best trials - best in the sense that they minimise the chance of bias in allocation, response or assessment of response, is a 'double-blind' trial, in which neither the patient or the investigator knows the true identity of the treatment until the study itself is completed, with all patients having completed all assessments. Such trials are frequently practical and ethical, and provision can always be made for the investigator to 'break the blind' - determine the identity of the treatment given to a specific patient - should it become clinically important to do so.

In some cases more sophisticated randomisation and blinding schemes are used, for example in cases where patients fall into distinct categories, e.g. according to disease stage, or some other prognostic factor. In those cases, simple randomisation schemes may need to be modified to produce 'stratified randomisation' whereby it is ensured that similar proportions of patients of each category are present in each of the possible treatment groups; it may or may not be necessary for patients and investigators to be kept unaware of the patient's stratification group.

Box 7.4 Trial design: the main options

Controls
- No control: avoid if possible
- Placebo: acceptable if no current standard therapy
- Active: desirable if a standard therapy exists (placebo may also be included)

Stopping rules
- Fixed sample: simple to design and analyses: may need more patients
- Interim analyses: use professional statistical help: may reduce required number of patients
- Sequential trial: use professional statistical help: may greatly reduce required number of patients.

Structure
- Parallel: should be preferred whenever possible
- Cross-over: use with caution

Blinding
- Open: avoid if possible
- Blind-at-randomisation: better than open!
- Single-blind: often acceptable with objective responses
- Double-blind: should be preferred whenever possible

Computer software for generation of randomisation codes is available.

Summary Clinical studies are best designed in a logical sequence of steps - though some iteration may be necessary as the design process proceeds. The steps are essentially: specify objectives; define the patient population; select control treatment; choose a trial structure; define a stopping rule; organise the randomisation and blinding scheme. Box 7.4 summarises the main options available. A more detailed summary of some of the topics discussed in this chapter can be found in Pocock (1983).

Further reading

- Brunier, H. and Whitehead, J. (1993). PEST - Planning and Evaluation of Sequential Trials - Operating Manual.
- Machin, D. and Campbell, M. J. (1993). Statistical tables for the design of clinical trials, 2nd ed. Oxford: Blackwell.
- Pocock, S.J. (1983). Clinical trials: a practical approach. Chichester: John Wiley and Sons.

- Whitehead, J. (1992). The design and analysis of sequential clinical trials. London: Ellis Horwood.
- European Agency for the Evaluation of Medicinal Products. (1998). Statistical Principles for Clinical Trials. ICH Topic E9. CPMP/ICH/363/96.
- European Agency for the Evaluation of Medicinal Products. (1998). General Considerations for Clinical Trials. ICH Topic E8. CPMP/ICH/291/195.

8

Data management and statistical analysis

Fiona Peachey and Les Huson

PART ONE: DATA MANAGEMENT

Introduction

The success of a clinical trial is dependent not only upon the design of a study protocol, but also upon the methods employed to ensure that clinical data are of high quality and in a suitable format for statistical analysis. These processes fall under the broad heading of 'data handling' and cover everything from data capture to monitoring, editing, database set-up, data entry, quality control and statistical analysis. A well designed data handling strategy will ensure the efficient collection and rapid processing of high quality clinical data. This chapter aims to give the reader a brief overview of some of key issues involved in these processes.

Data collection

Once a clinical trial has been designed, it is important to consider how best to collect the clinical information within a Case Report Form (CRF) or patient booklet. The design of a CRF is a critical factor in the capture of high quality data. Ideally a CRF should be well structured, easy to complete and specific enough to avoid the collection of unnecessary information. Two questions that need be addressed during this design process are: (1) why does this information need to be collected? and (2) how is it going to be analysed? If the answer to either of these questions is unclear from the study protocol or statistical analysis plan, the objectives of the study need to be reassessed and clarified. A common mistake in the design of CRFs is to collect too much information in the hope that some of it might be useful. Collection of extraneous and additional information serves only to take the emphasis away from the critical data, whilst it increases the amount of resource and time needed to collect, process and analyse the data.

The following two examples demonstrate the importance of having a well structured approach with specific questions. Two different formats have been used

Box 8.1 Medical History - 1

Give details of the patient's medical history ....
....
....

Box 8.2 Medical History - 2

Does the patient have a clinically significant medical history? Yes/No

If the answer to the above question is yes, complete details below:

Body system	Normal √	Abnormal √	Comments (if abnormal comment below)
Mental status			
Ears, eyes,nose, throat			
Cardiovascular system			
Respiratory system			
Central nervous system			
etc.			

Box 8.3 Herpes Zoster

Does the patient have clinically confirmed herpes zoster? Yes/No
- If yes, please complete details below:
  Date of onset of rash (d/m/y) __/__/__
  Time of onset of rash (00:00_24:00) __:__

Did the patient have prodromal pain? Yes/No
- If yes, complete the question below:
  Date of onset of prodromal pain (d/m/y) __/__/__

(Boxes 8.1 and 8.2) to collect the same information regarding the patients' medical history. The first example

(Box 8.1) uses a non-specific open ended question 'Give details of the patient's medical history ...., which allows the investigator to write as long or short a response as he/she wants in whatever format. In contrast the second example (Box 8.2) asks a specific closed question 'Does the patient have a clinically significant medical history Yes/No?' followed by a series of structured questions which only need to be completed if the answer to the initial header question is 'Yes'. Should the investigator indicate a particular body system as 'abnormal', he/she is then asked to provide further information in a specific 'Comments' section.

The major drawback with the example shown in Box 8.1 is the wide diversity of responses possible; this may vary from a complete blank response (does this mean no medical history?), to a single word, e.g. 'myocardial infarction' , to a lengthy paragraph, e.g. 'the patient had tight chest pains in 1996 and this was later diagnosed as a myocardial infarction'. In the last instance the critical information has to be filtered out from the paragraph, i.e. the abnormality is 'myocardial infarction' and the associated detail is '1996', this editing exercise can be both costly and inefficient. If the same information was collected in the format of the second example (Box 8.2), the investigator need only tick the 'cardiovascular' abnormality box and write 'myocardial infarction 1996' in the associated comment section. Thus the information is collected in a more standardised and optimised manner requiring minimal clarification or editing.

The collection of text should be avoided wherever possible and alternate methods sought for capturing this information. An investigator's handwriting will be notoriously bad, as is evident to anyone who has ever tried to read a prescription. Alternate formats could include using a pre-printed list of questions with a tick box, or using a series of structured or hierarchical questions (Box 8.3). This is especially important when dealing with large multicentre studies in countries where the language used in the CRF is not the primary language. This also promotes consistency of data capture and prevents the need for unnecessary data editing prior to data entry. There are, of course, some instances where the collection of text is unavoidable, e.g. the collection of adverse event terms.

A final point to consider during the design of any CRF

is whether this type of data is likely to be captured in future clinical trials, e.g. demography or physical examination data. If the answer is 'yes', every effort should be made to ensure that the same page layout is used for each trial to promote consistency of data capture and reporting.

Site education and training Depending upon the size and complexity of the clinical trial it may be necessary to provide the investigator(s) with some form of up front training or education explaining how the clinical trial should be managed; this should also include information regarding how the CRF should be completed (CRF Completion Guidelines). Site personnel training and specific workshops can organised to help investigators and study nurses get a better understanding of how/why data needs to be collected in a certain format. In addition, the use of written instructions (a Procedures manual) detailing everything from how to report a Serious Adverse Event to how to complete a particular CRF page can greatly assist an investigator during the trial period.

Data monitoring Data monitoring is a process that ensures the investigator is collecting complete, accurate and legible clinical data. Depending upon the size and complexity of a clinical trial, this process can take the format of a quick informal check of clinical trial data, e.g. 'Does the data make sense?' and 'Do the source documents match the data collected in the CRF?' to a detailed series of checks outlined in a document entitled 'Monitoring guidelines'. The latter document should aid the monitor through the process of monitoring and ensure that clinical data is as a complete, accurate and legible as possible before the CRF is removed from the investigator site. Identifying data queries at this stage of the data handling process is both time and resource efficient, since the investigator can verify and authorise changes/ corrections to the data immediately. It also serves to identify any parts of the CRF where the investigator is having a particularly difficult time filling in the CRF because he/she doesn't understand the question.

Data editing The process of data editing is one that ensures that the information collected in the CRF is in a suitable state for entry onto a clinical trial database. A typical example of editing is to highlight key words, e.g. 'myocardial infarction' in the previous example above, or alternatively reduce open text down to a set number of characters, e.g. 30 characters maximum. The reason for this process is twofold; firstly it reduces the time spent by data entry staff entering this information onto a database and secondly, data are collected on the database in a concise and easily reportable format. In this instance since text can only be listed, it cannot be analysed, it is beneficial to only enter critical data.

Editing may be largely redundant in cases where data have been well monitored. However, it is especially important when dealing with CRFs from a number of different investigator sites, which may have been monitored by a number of different individuals, i.e. a large multicentre study. In the latter case it helps to promote consistency and accuracy of data entry and identifies any missing or questionable data.

Clinical databases

Clinical data need to be captured in an organised format to facilitate reporting and analysis of data. This may take the format of a simple spreadsheet or a specialised trial-specific database. Whatever format is used, it is important that data is captured in such a way that it facilitates reporting and analysis, i.e. the statistician needs to perform minimal data manipulation and programming to complete the analysis.

Box 8.4 Grouped data

Scheduled time	Visit date	Zoster pain yes/no	Number of days with pain
Screen	02 Jan 1993	Y	7
Day 7	09 Jan 1993	Y	7
Day 14	16 Jan 1993	Y	5
Day 21	23 Jan 1993	N	0
Day 28	01 Feb 1993	Y	4
Follow-up	05 Jul 1993	Y	32

Figure 8.1 shows a typical example of the transfer of data from a CRF onto a database and its conversion into a format that allows easy analysis and reporting. This

Figure 8.1 Transfer of data to a database

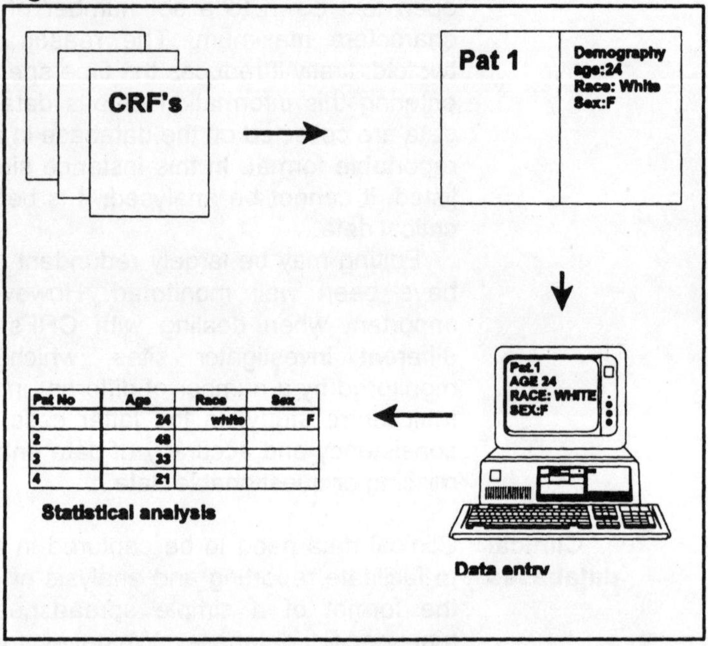

system utilises a relational database language, such as Progress or Oracle. The data are stored in a series of discrete tables depending upon the type of data, e.g. demographic, safety or efficacy data, and the statistician may 'join' tables to facilitate reporting. This type of data collection requires considerable planning up front during database design to ensure that data are reported in logical groups. Box 8.4 shows a typical example of this where the same data are collected over a series of time points. Although this occurs across a series of different CRF pages, the data are related to one another and therefore it makes more sense to group these data into a single table. Each 'row' of data represents information relating to a specific time point.

Regulatory requirements insist that whatever the system is used to capture and report clinical data, it must be fully tested and validated. The extent of validation required is not specified, however, it is necessary to demonstrate that data capture is accurate, reproducible and secure. It is also necessary to demonstrate some form of quality control and /or quality assurance.

Data entry Data entry, i.e. entering the clinical data onto a computer, may take one of several formats depending upon the requirements of the data entry system. Data may be entered once, twice or verified. In the first instance as the term suggests 'once' represents single entered data. Data entered twice are dual-entered, i.e. duplicate databases are set up and two entry operators enter identical data, the system that automatically compares the two versions and highlights any discrepancies for correction. The third version is key-over-key verification; this process is intermediate between the other two options, i.e. it involves a first entry of data, followed by a second entry operator re-entering data and correcting data immediately when a difference between the two versions is highlighted. Choosing the right form of data entry will depend upon the sophistication of the system being used, the type of person entering the data and the likelihood of key stroke errors. For example if a non-medically trained person is entering the data, it would be wise to use either dual data entry or key-over-key verification. On the other hand, someone who is very familiar with the data and medical terms, should have no problem entering the data only once, although given enough data to be entered such a person will also make errors.

Data quality control/ assurance

Data quality control refers to the process whereby the data on the database is checked for completeness, accuracy and consistency. Any rogue or missing data should be highlighted during this process and wherever possible corrected before statistical analysis. This process may be either performed manually or electronically depending upon the sophistication of the data entry system. Typical examples of quality control checks include:

- Identifying any missing critical data, i.e. efficacy or safety data
- Checking for consistency of responses, e.g. the response to a header question followed by the absence or presence of data
- Checking the completeness of dates and logical order

With larger databases, it is advisable to generate a Data Quality Control Strategy plan up front detailing exactly which types of data will be checked and to what level of detail.

Data Quality Assurance refers to the process whereby

the quality of the data captured on the database is compared to the clinical data captured within a CRF, i.e. the quality of the data entry and quality control processes. Usually a random sample of data on the database, e.g. 10%, is checked against the equivalent CRF pages and the number of errors found expressed as percentage error rate. Providing the data on the database is within an acceptable error rate, e.g. no more than 10 errors in 20,000 data fields, the overall data quality is acceptable and the database can be passed onto the statistician for analysis. Data quality assurance should be the last step performed before the data is handled over to the statistician for analysis.

PART TWO: STATISTICAL ANALYSIS

Statistical analysis plan

Long before a quality assured clinical database is delivered for statistical analysis, a statistical analysis plan should have been prepared; early drafts of this plan will, in fact, often be of considerable value during the construction and quality checking of the database.

A statistical analysis plan is simply a detailed description of the ways in which the data collected during the clinical study will be presented and analysed. It expands considerably on the plans outlined in the study protocol, which should be reasonably general in nature. A detailed statistical analysis plan has a number of uses. Firstly, it sets out in writing the proposed treatment of study data, so that all personnel connected with conduct of the study have an opportunity to review the plan, to comment on it, and contribute to it. Secondly, it allows professional statisticians and programmers to begin organising the production of data analyses and the associated computer programs at an early stage of database construction. Thirdly, the plan will help during the design and construction of the trial database, since it will specify how particular items of data are to be analysed, and therefore how they would best be stored in and accessed from the database. Finally, the existence of a written statistical analysis plan helps to demonstrate to external reviewers, that statistical analyses were planned in advance of inspection of the data, and hence are not the result of 'data dredging'. Analyses planned in advance in this way have considerably greater persuasive value. In preparing a statistical analysis plan, it helps to bear in mind the different categories of data that are typically collected in a clinical study; the proposed treatment of each category of data should be described in the plan. Box 8.5 lists some suggested categories; others may be appropriate in some studies. Statistical analysis of the trial

Box 8.5 Categories of data collected in clinical studies

- Demographic data
- Pre-treatment medical history and pre-treatment disease state
- Data on prognostic factors
- Dosing and exposure data
- Efficacy measurements
- Adverse event data
- Vital signs data
- Haematology and clinical chemistry results
- Other safety data, e.g. ECG, EEG
- Health economic data
- Other routine data on clinical care and monitoring

data will require the adoption of different approaches for the different categories.

Statistical approach to analysis

Much of the data collected in clinical studies can adequately be presented simply by using appropriate tables and/or graphical illustrations of simple summary statistics such as mean values, median values, minima, maxima, and standard deviations. Some types of data - especially efficacy data - will normally also be subject to more formal and technical analysis, using statistical significance tests and confidence intervals. The more important measures of safety should be summarised using confidence intervals.

Demographic data

The main reasons for collecting demographic data are to

- Describe the patients recruited into the study and
- To check that there are no great differences between those recruited into the different treatment groups.

A suitable summary of demographic data would be tabulation of the mean, median, minimum, maximum, standard deviation, and number of patients, for each quantitative measurement collected - such as age, body weight, height, surface area etc. If categorical data are collected e.g. race, sex, then the numbers and percentages of patients in each of the categories should be tabulated. These summaries should be presented overall, and separately for each of the treatment groups.

Statistical significance tests should *not* be used to compare the values between the different treatment groups.

Pre-treatment medical history and pre-treatment disease state Pre-treatment medical history and information on the disease state prior to treatment are both collected for the same reasons as demographic data: primarily to characterise the patients. Data in this category should be presented using the same techniques as those applied to demographic data.

Data on prognostic factors Prognostic factors identifiable in a patient prior to administration of treatment should also be presented using techniques similar to those applied to demographic data. However, since these factors are known to potentially affect the patient's response, it is good practice to examine the relationship between these factors and some or all of the efficacy measures. If the prognostic factors are categorical in nature (e.g. patients classified as smokers/non-smokers) then a suitable approach might be to summarise the main efficacy measure for each of the categories. With continuous quantitative prognostic factors (e.g. blood pressure), graphical analysis or regression analysis of the relationship between the factor and the efficacy variable might be appropriate.

Dosing and exposure data It is difficult to generalise about how dosing and exposure data should be summarised, since dosing regimes differ greatly from one drug to another. Often, it is desirable to summarise the modal doses received by patients during the course of a study, since these will typically be more representative of the treatment administered than statistics such as the mean or median, especially if some form of dose-escalation or tapering is part of the normal course of treatment. Overall duration of exposure to drug is also generally reported. In cases where there is a strong relationship between dose and response, and where a range of doses have been used in the study, some summary of the nature of the dose-response curve would be appropriate.

Efficacy measurements Formal statistical techniques will normally be used to analyse efficacy data. These will include statistical significance tests, with reporting of associated *p* values, and computation of confidence intervals estimating the magnitude of possible treatment effects. The number of formal statistical techniques available is large; Box 8.6 summarises some of the main types of efficacy measurement that might be used, and the more obvious techniques associated with analysis of such measurements.

Box 8.6 Typical efficacy endpoints and associated statistical techniques

Values of continuous measurement (e.g. blood pressure)

- if measurements are normally distributed: T-tests and associated confidence intervals to compare two mean values; analysis of variance to compare three or more.
- if measurements have a non-normal distribution: Wilcoxon rank tests with confidence intervals for medians

Comparing proportions of patients responding to a treatment

- Chi-squared or binomial tests with associated confidence intervals
  or
- Relative risks and associated confidence intervals

Survival data (or time-to-event data)

- Logrank statistics, with graphical presentation of Kaplan-Meier survival curves, and tabulation of summaries such as median time-to-event.
  or
- Cox proportional-hazard regression model.

Adverse event data

In most cases 'safety' data such as adverse event reports are collected with the hope of demonstrating that the test treatment is no different from the control. This is based upon an entirely different hypothesis from that proposed for efficacy data, where the objective is generally to show that there *is* a difference between test and control. Because the objective of collecting safety data is different, the approach to analysis must also be varied. In particular, it is rarely appropriate to use statistical significance tests to analyse safety data. A significance test is a tool that can be used to help to establish if an difference between treatments is likely to be real. It *cannot* be used to demonstrate that two treatments are similar in their effects. The only exception to this rule would be in a situation where it is specified *in advance* - in the statistical analysis plan - that a difference between two treatments is possible in respect of the rate of some particular adverse event, and that a significance test will be used to investigate this possibility.

More usually, the best approach to analysis of adverse event data and other 'safety' data, is to present suitable summary statistics, together with confidence intervals. In the case of adverse event data, the rate of occurrence of each distinct adverse event on each treatment group should be reported, together with confidence intervals for the difference between rates of occurrence on the different treatments. An alternative would be to present risk ratios or 'relative risks' of occurrence, with confidence intervals for the relative risk.

Haematology and clinical chemistry data

A summary of median values will generally be useful for most haematology and chemistry measurements, since these tend not to have symmetrical distributions. The laboratory used to assay these variables will have established 'normal' or 'reference' ranges for each of the measurements, which purport to specify the limits within which most values will lie. The implication is that any value outside of the 'reference' range might have some clinical significance, and might be worth examining in more detail. It will therefore usually be helpful to summarise the numbers and percentages of reported values which fall above and below the upper and the lower limits of the appropriate reference range, using different ranges for the different sexes or for different age groups or races, as appropriate. However, a change over time of one of these values within the normal range may be just as important and graphical representation over time will reveal this.

Health economic data

As the costs of providing health care continue to rise rapidly, more and more assessments of new therapies are starting to include an evaluation of the costs and benefits associated with the application of a particular treatment. The methods of analysis of such data are extensive and specialised, and it will generally be advisable to seek professional advice from a health economist before analysis of anything other than the simplest cost data.

Other data collected during routine clinical care

During most trials, other incidental items of data may be collected during the normal process of clinical care of a patient, or during monitoring of a study. The final report of a trial should include a description of any such ancillary items of data, and anything of particular clinical significance will naturally be discussed. Otherwise, it will be sufficient either to provide a simple listing of such data, or at least to have a listing available for inspection by anyone who will review the final trial report.

Further reading

- Altman, D.G. (1991). Practical statistics for medical research. London: Chapman and Hall.
- European Agency for the Evaluation of Medicinal Products. (1998). Statistical Principles for Clinical Trials. ICH Topic E9. CPMP/ICH/363/96.
- European Agency for the Evaluation of Medicinal Products. (1998). General Considerations for Clinical Trials. ICH Topic E8. CPMP/ICH/291/195.

Other data collected during routine clinical care

During most trials, other incidental items of data may be collected during the normal process of clinical care of a patient, or during monitoring of a study. The final report of a trial should include a description of any such ancillary items of data and anything of particular clinical significance will generally be discussed. Otherwise, it will be sufficient either to provide a simple listing of such data, or at least to have a listing available for inspection by anyone who will review the final trial report.

Further reading

- Altman, D.G. (1991). Practical statistics for medical research. London: Chapman and Hall.
- European Agency for the Evaluation of Medicinal Products. (1998). Statistical Principles for Clinical Trials. ICH Topic E9. CPMP/ICH/363/96.
- European Agency for the Evaluation of Medicinal Products. (1998). General Considerations for Clinical Trials. ICH Topic E8. CPMP/ICH/291/95.

9

Ethical considerations

Gregor Jemec and Patricia Sohl

Ethics is the branch of philosophy that deals with values relating to human conduct. Ethics is concerned with concepts such as good or bad. These concepts are ubiquitous elements of human life, and are therefore also present in the pursuit of knowledge through science. Medical ethics is the application of philosophical knowledge to the doctor - patient relationship in order to promote the patients health and subsequent autonomy.

Basic principles

Gillon has produced a very useful summary of medical ethics giving four moral principles that are relatively independent of personal philosophy, politics or religion, based on the work by Beauchamp and Childress. These are

- **Principle I: Respect for autonomy**
  Respect for the autonomy of others has many implications in medical research. It is the basis for obtaining agreement before involving subjects in an experiment, but also for confidentiality.
- **Principle II: Beneficence ('Doing good')**
  and
- **Principle III: Non-maleficence ('Not doing harm')**
  When there is a risk of harming patients when trying to help them principles II and III are considered together with the aim to produce more benefit than harm. There are also cases when the principles are separated, for example when healthy volunteers are studied and no benefit can be expected. Non-maleficence is then the only concern.
- **Principle IV: Justice**
  This principle in general relates to fairness and involves respect for morally acceptable laws, people's rights and distribution of scarce resources.

Ethics play a role in our assessment of scientific matters,

and the four principles indicated above may help to give structure to these considerations.

Ethics and clinical drug research - importance of autonomy

Clinical science is by definition carried out with other human beings. Human subjects are by definition self-determining persons, and this means that normal ethical considerations in terms of rights and obligations have to be respected, as in any other interpersonal relationship. The concept of self determination or autonomy can be considered as the backbone of most ethical systems and is important in clinical research. The physician facilitates the practice of autonomy by the patient by reducing the dependence caused by disease.

Since its articulation by Hume, a basic principle of democratic societies is that human beings have a value in and of themselves, that is to say, they must be protected simply because they are human beings, and cannot be used as a means to another person's end. A derivative principle of this rule is that human beings must themselves agree to what they will or will not participate in. In society in general this is reflected by common legal requirements for, e,g. veracity in commerce, the foundations of all commercial law. In relations between humans it is important to realise that moral principles often have a substantial non-rational value to us as human beings. This is most easily illustrated by the difference between comfort about telling an insignificant lie - and the related discomfort when discovering that we have been told a lie, i.e. when we have been used for someone's purpose. This non-rational or emotional aspect is especially important in situations where professional ethics apply.

In the conduct of a clinical trial the investigator has to take into account several levels of ethical considerations and obligations, which all stem from the basic respect for individual self-determination and autonomy.

Clinical research involves physicians and patients. An additional level of professional ethical considerations is therefore added. Professions traditionally have developed around specific areas of expertise and a monopoly in the exercise thereof. Two classic examples of professions are clergy and medicine. Other members of society are dependent on this expert knowledge, and professions are therefore generally granted high levels of autonomy within society. Professional ethics confirm basic social moral principles of interhuman activities, and in cases where professions have the power to injure or constrain the expression of self-determination, the ethics of the profession is often expressed as a code (eg. the Hippocratic Oath) and act as a guarantee to society that these powers will only be used to serve the best interests of fellow human beings. Physicians are granted clinical autonomy by society, which can be expressed as the freedom to choose what is best for the patient, but this is only granted on the condition that the patient's best interests are served. The special knowledge of the professions therefore impose extra ethical obligations on them.

The Helsinki Declaration: Basic principles for clinical research

Following the atrocities of the Second World War, both physicians and societies have paid more attention to the protection of individual self-determination and autonomy. The first set of moral principles guiding medical research was expressed in the Nurenberg Code after the trials against Nazi concentration camp doctors. Subsequently this has been outlined in greater detail in the so called Helsinki Declaration (see Box 9.1), although it has been modified numerous times in other places since its conception in 1964 and the latest version is from 1989 and modified in Hong Kong. The four principles of medical ethics referred to above can be found back in the Declaration.

The key elements of the declaration are:

- Scientific design
- A risk-benefit evaluation
- Informed consent
- Independent review

Scientific design

Scientific design is one of the themes of this book. In ethical terms scientific design is important because a good design is a prerequisite for any risk-benefit evaluation and hence for informed consent. Good scientific design will allow the researcher to answer a relevant question with a minimum risk to his fellow human beings. Literature review, sample size and statistical analysis are all necessary in order to evaluate risk, to minimize exposure and to avoid superfluous re-exposure of human subjects. Bad science in its most extreme, exposes human subjects to unnecessary risk of no benefit to anyone.

Research involving humans must be based upon accepted scientific principles and laboratory and animal experimentation.

- Each study should be described in a protocol and considered by an independent review committee.
- Studies should be conducted by scientifically qualified personnel and supervised by a medically qualified person, who has final responsibility. Responsibility can never be transferred to the subject, even if the subject has given consent.
- The importance of the objective must be in proportion to the risk to the subject.
- The interests of the subject must prevail over those of society. Predictable risks must be balanced against foreseeable benefits to the subject and others.
- Special attention must be given to privacy and minimising the impact of the study on the integrity of the subject.
- Research should only be performed if the hazards are believed to be predictable. If the hazards outweigh the benefits in a study it should be stopped.
- Accurate publication is mandatory. Reports that do not comply with the declaration should not be published.
- Freely given informed consent should be obtained preferably in writing. The subjects will be informed that they may leave the study at any time without consequences.
- Subjects should not be dependent on the physician obtaining informed consent.
- When subjects are physically or mentally incompetent to give consent this should be obtained from relatives or legal guardians. When a minor child is able to give consent this must be obtained in addition to that of the legal guardian.
- The protocol should always contain an ethical statement and should state that the principles from this declaration are complied with.

For the full text refer to:

Declaration of Helsinki

- 18th World Medical Assembly, Helsinki, Finland (June 1964)

- 29th World Medical Assembly, Tokyo, Japan (October 1975)
- 35th World Medical Assembly, Venice, Italy (October 1983)
- 41st World Medical Assembly, Hong Kong (September 1989)

Risk and benefit

Risk and benefit are core elements of any ethical analysis. In order for society and individuals to accept the inevitable risks associated with clinical trials, an element of motivation is necessary. Motivation can be derived from many different levels of abstraction, i.e. physical, individual or societal motivation. It is important to notice here, that risk and benefit are not necessarily at the opposite ends of a spectrum for the individual human subject. For example the use of untested substances in the treatment of AIDS certainly has risks and sometimes benefits for the individual, but offers society different benefits for example through information on toxicity. However, the principle of autonomy would prevent the use of human beings for obtaining this information unless net benefit for *the individual* is obtained. This therefore involves the full disclosure of any and all mortal risks to the patient no matter what their likelihood. The patient may subsequently be advised about the relative probability of the risks.

Informed consent

The two former subjects are discussed extensively in this book and - although they can often give rise to ethical disputes - can generally be resolved. In many cases a more common point of ethical contention is that of informed consent, which is why this will receive special attention.

Informed consent is a procedure, not a finished product, and the fact that a signed consent form exists does not mean that informed consent has taken place. The procedure is intended to provide the basis for a fully informed choice by a self-determining autonomous person, and all requirements are intended to safeguard the autonomy of the individual. From this it is also clear, that human subjects can withdraw their consent at any point during the study.

The reader is invited to entertain the communication model in which the relationship is defined as sender - receiver in order to analyse the possible pitfalls of communication. Problems may occur with the formulation of the message at the sender, in transmission, or with the receiver's understanding of the message.

Communication problems are not always due to the sender, but the responsibilities of sender and receiver are different, e.g. the sender is responsible for the formulation of the message, while the receiver is responsible for the decoding, and each of these processes offer opportunity for insufficient communication. There is therefore not only ample examples of insufficient attention being paid to the formulation of information, but also of patients either not understanding or suppressing any recollection of information given. This may particularly occur when other major events, such as e.g. major surgery, cloud the attention of the patient.

Informed consent must be:

- Informative
- Understandable
- Free
- Competent

Informative The information must contain all necessary data to make it possible for human subjects to come to a decision. All side-effects with a potentially fatal outcome must be listed. It is important to realise that the obligation to inform a subject of a potential side-effect of a trial is independent of the chance of this side-effect occurring. The decision to accept or reject a given risk is strictly personal and cannot be generalised. In practical terms it is necessary for the investigator not only to be knowledgable about the subject of the study, but also about the reasons for writing the consent and the type of patient or subject who reads it. This may require the help of another person not involved in research and not involved in the trial at hand. Most human subjects will have difficulty in determining the significance of the risks and benefits described in the informed consent for their personal situation.

Understandable Structuring the information in an appropriate way is usually a difficult task for most investigators. The writing must be clear, simple and brief, accurate and complete, polite and human. This sounds self-evident, but is more difficult to achieve than many investigators would care to admit. Inspiration for the text can be derived from instructions for the use of household goods, the tabloid press and advertising. The key elements are simplicity and brevity. Use short words, not long words. Use short sentences, not long sentences. Simple words are better than complicated foreign words. Several re-writes are usually necessary to construct a good information sheet, and at all times attention must be paid to the contents, so as not to reduce the informative value of the writing as it is simplified. The standard consent form does not exist. The content does depend on the background of the subjects, the type of trial and most likely the country in which the trial is performed. Nevertheless all consent forms should comply with the basic principles indicated in this chapter.

Free Absence of coercion is a prerequisite for valid consent, this is the case in contract law as well as informed consent. Unintended coercion can take place in many ways. Time is a factor, and human subjects must have sufficient time to consider their participation in a drug trial. No fixed rules can be given, but 24 hours will suffice in most cases where this delay is practical. In the clinical environment there are other possibilities for unintended coercion, which physicians are not always fully aware of. Participation in a trial must not in any way compromise future treatment. This may seem obvious, but is often a latent fear in patients. It is therefore useful that the attending physician is not the person to perform the informed consent procedure. He or she may however freely answer any questions, and should at all times confirm that no matter which decision the patient comes to regarding the trial, this will have no influence whatsoever on their treatment and care. Whenever a potential state of dependency exists between the human subjects and the investigators, e.g. employees or students, similar care must be taken to ensure that consent is given freely.

Competent Finally, consent must be competent to be valid. The consent of a two-year old is invalid. The person must understand the consequences of the consent. In some areas of research this element causes genuine problems, for example in paediatrics, obstetrics or psychiatry. In these cases substituted consent can be used. Substituted consent is consent given by a family member or guardian on behalf of the incompetent human subject. Substituted consent is an inferior solution, different from true informed consent for obvious reasons. The substituted consent attempts to secure individual autonomy through a paternalistic procedure in which a guardian is appointed. The guardian can estimate risk independently and can promote benefit, but cannot by the very nature of the relationship promote autonomy which is the core of informed consent.

As can be seen from the preceding paragraphs the informed consent process requires the mastering of several steps to function properly. It does however, offer the investigator the benefits not only of ethical behaviour, access to journals which will publish the results, trouble-free interaction with the ethical committee, etc., but also more tangible benefits for the trial at hand. The informed consent enables you to motivate the human subjects and secures their enthusiastic collaboration in the study, because they fully understand what they have agreed to.

Guidelines for the informed consent form

Both in the USA and in Europe clear rules exist about informed consent and any aspiring clinical researcher should read the relevant sections in the Good Clinical Practice regulations (two pages-relevant to Europe) and the Food and Drug Administration regulations (about four pages-relevant to the USA). The Food and Drug regulations stipulate which elements should be present in any consent form (see Box 9.2).

Independent review

The ethical committee or the Institutional Review Board embodies the procedures required by the Helsinki Declaration and the different regulations in Europe and the USA. The actual organization of these committees may differ from country to country, and there is no evidence for linking one particular type of organization or procedure with performance. In addition to any specific national rules and regulations which may exist in this area, it is more a question of understanding the role of the ethical committee and structuring the organization to fulfil this role. The role of the ethical committee is to evaluate a planned study in terms of its ethical aspects, and thereby promote the interests of society and protect the autonomy of individuals in general.

These committees must therefore meet certain basic membership requirements. The development of democracy has generally required that non-professionals determine the non-expertise elements of any decision. The committees must therefore contain experts as well as non-expert members in a balanced way. In addition the committees must meet basic bureaucratic requirements for a functioning body: a definition of the quorum, defined procedures and appropriate record keeping. In some countries the committees are also asked to perform a continuing review of ongoing research, in which case it may be necessary to form subcommittees.

Basic elements

In seeking informed consent, the following information shall be provided to each subject:

1. a) A statement that the study involves research
   b) An explanation of the purposes of research
   c) The expected duration of the subject's participation
   d) A description of the procedures to be followed and
   e) Identification of any procedures which are experimental.
2. A description of any reasonably foreseeable risks or discomforts to the subject.
3. A description of any benefits to the subject or others which may reasonably be expected from the research.
4. A disclosure of appropriate alternative procedures or courses of treatment, if any, that may be advantageous to the subject.
5. a) A statement describing the extent, if any, to which confidentiality of records identifying the subject will be maintained and
   b) A notification that the Food and Drug Administration (or another regulatory body if applicable) may inspect the records.
6. a) For research involving more than minimal risk, an explanation as to whether any compensation and an explanation as to whether any treatments are available if injury occurs and, if so, what they consist of or
   b) where further information may be obtained.
7. An explanation of whom to contact for answers to pertinent questions about the research and research subjects' rights and whom to contact in the event of a research-related injury to the subject.
8. a) A statement that participation is voluntary
   b) that refusal to participate will involve no penalty or loss of benefits to which the subject is otherwise

entitled and

c) that the subject may discontinue participation at any time without penalty or loss of benefits to which the subject is otherwise entitled.

Additional elements When appropriate, one or more of the following elements of information shall also be provided to each subject:

1. A statement that the particular treatment or procedure may involve risks to the subject (or to the embryo or fetus), which are currently unforeseeable.
2. Anticipated circumstances under which the subject's participation may be terminated by the investigator without regard to the subject's consent.
3. Any additional costs to the subject that may result from participation in the research.
4. The consequences of a subject's decision to withdraw from the research and procedures for orderly termination by the subject.
5. A statement that significant new findings developed during the course of the research which may relate to the subject's willingness to continue participation will be provided to the subject.
6. The approximate number of subjects involved in the study.

If you are in a position where you have to set up an ethical review system the reference material indicated at the end of this chapter will give you guidance. The FDA regulations are explicit about the details of the process and this should be a good starting point. Obviously local laws will determine what needs to be done as well.

Ethical considerations are necessary in all clinical trials. The guiding principle is the promotion of self-determination and autonomy for the human subjects involved. This is done through the appropriate design of relevant studies, which take into account the risks as well as the benefits for not only the individual but society as well. A system of ethical committees should be organised to help investigators monitor the ethical aspects of any trials. Investigators should always check the national professional regulations and rules before submitting protocols.

Wait for approval from the ethical committee before starting the study. It is mandatory that studies are conducted only following fully informed consent. The process of informed consent requires the investigator to communicate the risks and benefits of a proposed study to the human subjects, who then freely and without any coercion give their consent. This can only be achieved without conflict if sufficient attention is paid to the clarity and contents of the information given. Investigators should furthermore remember that the ethical process is not as much an obstacle to research, as an additional effort to ensure the quality of science.

Further reading

- Beauchamp TL, Childress JF. (1983) Principles of biomedical ethics. 2nd edition. New York: Oxford University Press.
- Brody, H. (1981). Ethical decisions in medicine. Boston: Little, Brown & Co.
- Gillon, R. (1994). Medical ethics: Four principles plus attention to scope. British Medical Journal 309: 184-188.
- Katz, J., ed. (1972). Experimentation with human beings. New York: Russel Sage.
- Silberman, W. M. (1975). Human experimentation: A guided step into the unknown. Oxford: Oxford University Press.

References

- Good clinical practice for trials on medicinal products in the European Community. EEC Note for Guidance. III/3976/88 -EN (1.7.1991).
- Food and Drug Administration. Title 21 Food and Drugs, Part 50: Protection of human subjects, Subpart B: Informed consent of human subjects.
- Food and Drug Administration. Title 21 Food and Drugs, Part 56: Institutional review board, Subpart B: Organisation and personnel; Subpart C: IRB functions and operations; Subpart D: Records and reports.
- US Department of Health, Education and Welfare. The Belmont Report. Ethical principles and guidelines for the protection of human subjects of research. Bethesda, MD: National Institutes of Health, Office for Protection from Research Risks.

Appendix: Example of an informed consent form

Reference numbers in brackets refer to Box 9.2 (Elements of informed consent) demonstrating how you can evaluate your own informed consent form against this checklist.

You are in hospital, because you have heartburn. You also have undergone a gastroscopy - a test during which your doctor has looked into your stomach through a tube. This has demonstrated that the acid from your stomach - which caused the heartburn has slightly damaged the tube through which the food enters your stomach (the esophagus).

Studies on animals have shown the drug Sana to be a good new treatment of heartburn. In this research project [1a] we are trying to see if Sana helps against the damage to the esophagus [1b] and if it does this better than the drugs we usually give to patients. This study may help to provide information about which drug may treat this condition best at the lowest possible cost [3].

Half of all the patients in our study will receive the new drug Sana in a dose of 50 mg per day. The other half will receive the standard treatment that is usually given for this condition called omeprazole in a dose of 20 mg per day [4]. All patients fill in a form every morning in which they tell us how much heartburn they have. You do not have to give any blood samples in this study. You will have to take tablets and fill in the forms for a period of three weeks [1c, 1d]. A the end of this period you have to return to hospital and will undergo another gastroscopy. This test would have been performed regardless if you participate in this study or not [1e].

If people know they are getting a new drug, they may think it works better. We draw lots for who gets Sana, and who gets the standard treatment. You will not know if you are getting Sana or standard treatment, and neither will your doctor. All tablets have a code, and at the end of the study we can tell you which pill you got.

Sana has been tested on healthy people. Two out of 275 got a rash which may have to do with taking Sana. The rash went away after treatment. One person out of 275 got a fever and jaundice, which went away after treatment. None of the side-effects was serious [2].

If you want to know which pill you got, tell us and we will send you the information when the study is complete.

Remember that if you want to stop being part of the study you are free to do so at any time. If you decide not to participate or to get out of the study you will get the same treatment as before [8abc].

Any personal data we collect about you will of course be kept fully confidential. It is however possible that medical personnel from the Pharmaceutical Company involved in this research may see your records or that the governmental agency will see these during an inspection [5ab].

If you want more information about this study please ask your doctor or call dr Curious on telephone number 89 123 456 [7].

I declare that the contents of this form were explained to me on ________ in the presence of dr ________ and that I have read and understood this information.

Date ________ Patients signature

10

Aspects of study conduct

Steve Warrington

Introduction

Even if the ethics, design, protocol and planning of a clinical research study have been considered thoroughly, and preparation is immaculate, there remains a substantial risk that the project will fail because of shortcomings in the actual conduct of the work. Problems may arise at any stage, and the following guidance clearly cannot cover all eventualities; the aim is to alert you to the most common pitfalls and to suggest both prophylactic and remedial measures.

Recruitment

Patients

There are never enough patients for a clinical drug research study. The most serious shortfalls tend to arise when the protocol demands 'new' or 'treatment naive' patients: the quality of family practitioners is now generally high, and most patients receive some appropriate treatment before referral to the clinic. Even previously-treated patients seem to become scarce as soon as the trial begins.

The best approach to this problem is to avoid it by undertaking to study only a few patients, probably as part of a multi-centre trial, but unfortunately clinicians almost invariably overestimate the size of their pool of eligible subjects. Various remedies may be tried.

- **Advertisement**
  There are usually ethical, professional and scientific objections to the recruitment of patients by general advertisement. 'Patients with poorly-controlled high blood pressure required for trial of new medicine', or even 'Gloomy for no good reason? You could help yourself, and other victims of depression, by trying out a new medicine at your local hospital', would raise a few eyebrows in both lay and medical communities. However, advertisement may be appropriate when the condition of interest is a minor one for which patients usually do not seek medical advice. 'Sufferers from

cold sores needed for trial of new ointment - call 123 4567 the moment you feel one coming on' would surely be acceptable, as might 'Always getting athlete's foot? Help us test a new treatment' or 'Volunteers wanted for a trial of a new medicine for hay fever'. If you do recruit patients by advertisement, you should inform the family practitioner so that the individual's suitability for the study can be confirmed.

Several modes of advertisement are available at little or no cost. Postcard- or A4-sized notices may be distributed to local libraries, businesses and educational institutions, with permission where necessary. Local newspapers may be willing to publish an article about your project. You could ask the Teletext TV services (Ceefax and Oracle in the UK) to display an appeal in their 'voluntary services' sections, but these will be distributed nation-wide rather than just locally. If you are obliged to pay commercial rates for any advertisement, the pharmaceutical sponsor will usually be happy to bear the costs rather than see their project stalled through lack of eligible patients - but do be sure to consult them before incurring unbudgeted expenses. Increasingly internet websites are used for recruitment of patients or volunteers.

There is an important place for advertising if you are seeking patients with a rare condition. In that circumstance, you might consider asking a medical journal to publish an appeal to other clinicians to refer their patients. Success is more likely if the condition is untreatable as well as being rare.

- **Patient database**

The near-universal availability of personal computers has given the clinician the ability to maintain a database of patients classified by diagnosis or any other relevant feature. Suitable subjects for a study can be identified by appropriate interrogation of the database, and the patients invited to attend the clinic to discuss their possible participation. This procedure can only be used if the computer system has been established well before the study begins; setting up the database is too lengthy a task to be used as a salvage measure once recruitment has started. An established system could also be used to estimate the likely number of eligible patients before the investigator gives a commitment to undertake the study. The availability of patient databases means that it is no longer acceptable to ask outpatients to attend the clinic at regular but infrequent intervals in case they might be needed for a research project. In truth, such a practice was never acceptable.

- **Hospital colleagues**
  Asking senior clinical colleagues to refer patients eligible for your study does not work. It is hard enough to recruit patients for your own study, but it is almost impossible to summon the energy to recruit patients for someone else. However, you should certainly consider asking your junior medical staff to help; they can be extremely effective in finding patients.

- **Local family practitioners**
  If you are seeking patients with a common condition, particularly one that does not normally justify referral to a hospital clinic, writing to local family practitioners may be worth a try. A good response is more likely if there is no satisfactory established treatment for the condition. Sometimes it may be better to ask family practitioners to display notices in their surgery waiting rooms rather than to identify and refer suitable patients themselves.

  Irrespective of your choice of methods of increasing the recruitment of patients into your study, it is vital that you take rapid action if recruitment rates are inadequate. The best advice is 'Panic early' rather than 'Don't panic'. Remember that your data may be devalued or unusable if you study fewer patients than the minimum block size (see Chapter 7).

Healthy volunteers

Recruiting healthy volunteers is much easier than finding patients eligible for a study, but serious shortages can still occur - particularly if you have rarely or never used volunteer subjects previously, or if the study is very demanding of time and effort on the subject's part. Possible sources of volunteers are:

- **Your own department**
  At one time studies were small enough to be completed using volunteers from a single department only. Now, however, a minimum of 12 subjects is the norm and the net must be cast wider. If you do use any members of

your own department, you must be aware of the ethical difficulties of this practice (see Chapter 9).

- **Your hospital/college**
Teaching hospitals each have a few thousand staff, but displaying notices appealing for volunteers will probably yield only a handful of responses. Many other departments are competing for a share of that small number of individuals who are willing to contemplate participation in a research study. Nevertheless, local advertisement is quick and easy, and forms a useful part of the recruitment campaign - especially in a non-teaching hospital. Your notices should be informative enough to prevent ineligible or unsuitable subjects wasting their time (and yours) by responding. You should mention that payment will be made for the time and inconvenience of participation, but the amount should not be specified unless you also make clear exactly what participants will have to do.
  Do not make direct approaches to students or junior staff; it is impossible to exclude an element of coercion, benign though you may believe your public image to be. However, if you already have students or staff acting as your volunteers, it is acceptable to ask them to spread news of your project among their friends and colleagues.

- **Other institutions**
Placing notices in other teaching hospitals is worthwhile even though the yield from any one institution is unlikely to be great. You may get a better response from non-medical colleges because of the absence of competition from other departments. Be sure to obtain any permission necessary before displaying your notices. I have found this to be a problem only when seeking to advertise in the premises of large local businesses, perhaps because the occupational health officers feel too great a responsibility for their charges.

- **The community**
Unless you need only a few volunteers from time to time, you will almost certainly have to seek recruits in the community within a few miles of your institution. You can advertise for volunteers in the same ways as

for patients (see above), but it is often enough simply to ask your existing volunteers to spread the word to their friends and relations in the area. I have found 'word of mouth' to be consistently effective as a means of recruiting healthy young subjects. It is also salutary to know that your success depends on your reputation for looking after the volunteers well.

Middle-aged and elderly subjects may be difficult to recruit in large numbers, the middle-aged because they find it difficult to take time off work and the elderly because they are not attuned to the idea of medicines research. Wide advertisement may be needed to establish a 'panel' of potential volunteers. Once established, panels tend to be self-sustaining because the members recruit others on your behalf, often without prompting. However, panels tend to atrophy if they are not used regularly, so they work best in units that have a steady flow of research projects.

Do not forget to notify the family practitioner or student medical officer before the volunteer enters the study.

Consent

The ethical aspects of consent have been considered in Chapter 9, but some practical matters deserve consideration.

You must give the subjects written information about the study as this is now almost a universal legal requirement. In any case, you cannot conceivably describe the study clearly and comprehensively on 12 or more occasions, and the subjects cannot be expected to digest a detailed speech. Furthermore, an information sheet can be taken home, re-read and shown to others for advice and discussion. Whether you write the document yourself or use one supplied by the study sponsor, have it vetted by a non-medical person and defer to their views if they are critical. If you want to alter the sponsor's information sheet, tell them so before it has been finalised and agreed with any other study centres. If you really cannot accept a sheet that is already in use, the sponsor may be able to accommodate your idiosyncrasy but is unlikely to do so with enthusiasm.

Patients or volunteers sometimes ask to see the Investigators' Brochure or the study protocol, and you should allow them to do so. However, they cannot usually be allowed to take those documents away from the research unit, because of the sponsor's legitimate concerns about secrecy of commercially sensitive information.

Inclusion/ exclusion criteria

Ascertaining compliance with the inclusion/exclusion criteria is one of the least rewarding tasks in a research study, but it is also one of the most vital. In patient studies the criteria define the exact nature of the population to be tested, and deviation from them may later necessitate the exclusion of patients from the analysis of efficacy. This is not only scientifically undesirable but is also ethically unacceptable, since patients will have been subjected to inconvenience, and perhaps discomfort and risk of injury, in exchange for a benefit that is less than it should have been. Deviations from inclusion/exclusion criteria tend to be less frequent and serious in volunteer studies, mainly because the concept of a healthy subject is fairly uniform among clinicians. Nevertheless great care is needed in both patients and volunteers; unfortunately, some writers of protocols increase the risk of errors by giving banal or trivial criteria equal prominence with the most crucial ones.

If a particular criterion seems in practice to be impractical, unnecessary or unduly restrictive, the need for it should be discussed with the study sponsor. It is a simple matter to agree and issue a protocol amendment (see Chapter 6) altering the criteria, and other study centres may then also benefit from the changes.

Case report forms often contain a checklist that reflects most or all of the inclusion/exclusion criteria. Do not tick every box, mechanically, at the end of the interview and examination. Each question should be reviewed separately, and it is a good practice to ask the subject each one again. Remember that a single error at this stage can make all the rest of your work with that subject a waste of time.

Screening of patients and healthy volunteers

A screening procedure is essential in every study, not only to determine whether the subjects comply with the inclusion/ exclusion criteria but also to identify:

- features that might make the subjects' participation hazardous, such as a concurrent illness or risk factors for illness
- abnormalities that might later be attributed incorrectly

to the study medication

The minimum acceptable screening of patients or healthy volunteers comprises a clinical history and brief physical examination, similar to those used in screening applicants for life insurance. Haematology, biochemistry and urinalysis are regarded as essential in volunteers and are usually done in patients too. Additional specialised tests may be needed, particularly in patient studies. Any tests that are not part of the patient's routine care should be included in the budget for the study. Consult the appropriate departments before the study begins, and make sure they receive payment promptly.

Drugs of abuse

It is usual to test volunteers' urine for drugs of abuse such as cannabis, opiates, cocaine, amphetamines and benzodiazepines, but in my experience positive results are rare for all but cannabinoids. There is potential here for great embarrassment if you include colleagues, junior staff or students in your study, so try to avoid using them if possible. For no very obvious reason, patients are not usually subjected to screening for drugs of abuse; perhaps that will change in future.

Hepatitis B and C

Hepatitis B is very easily transmitted via blood, plasma or serum contamination of syringes, needles or fluids for injection. Volunteer studies nearly always include extensive blood sampling, and it is good practice to check that the subjects are negative for hepatitis B surface antigen (HBsAg) at the entry examination. Patients are not generally tested for HBsAg before they enter clinical drug studies, but there is little justification for this omission unless little or no blood sampling is to be done. You should offer vaccination against hepatitis B to all your staff who may be required to take or to handle blood samples. You should also notify them of the procedure to be followed if contamination incidents occur. Although hepatitis C may be less infectoious it is a common cause of chronic hepatitis and hence disturbance of liver biochemistry which, otherwise, may be attributed to the study drug.

HIV antibody

Ethical considerations have in the past prevented HIV antibody screening from becoming routine, but the greatly improved prognosis after multiple drug treatment will change this attitude. The need for counselling before the test also discourages clinicians from performing it. Nevertheless, volunteer studies in particular offer scope for transmission of infection because of the processing of multiple blood samples, and protocols are increasingly likely in future to specify that HIV testing should be done. The ethical implications of this require careful consideration also in view of new modes of treatment.

Informing the family practitioner You must notify the family practitioner of any important abnormalities that you find, whether the subject is a healthy volunteer or a patient. If the subject is not registered with a physician, direct referral to a hospital department may be necessary. Do not be tempted to assume responsibility for a volunteer's medical care.

Medical cover: nurses and physicians There is no substitute for carrying out the entire study yourself. No delegate can be as well-informed about the study or as meticulous as the principal investigator. However, a clinical drug study is a major undertaking and you will almost certainly need help from other physicians, or nurses or technicians. Choose your helpers carefully, and consider who is likely to do each job best. Research nurses are usually better than physicians at following instructions to the letter, and at keeping complete and accurate records; the physicians tend to be too improvisatory, and are inclined to ignore the protocol if its requirements do not fit with their preconceptions. Technicians excel with electrical and mechanical equipment, though some physicians come a close second. A physician is essential where there is a clinical need for one, but you must be certain that he or she is adequately trained to handle any emergencies that might arise. Not all physicians can confidently manage a cardiac catastrophe, for example.

When you allocate responsibility for part of the study, make clear whether it is acceptable for that responsibility to be further delegated if the need arises.

In some studies, it is preferable that all the main assessments are made by the same person. For example, psychiatric rating scales require training and experience if they are to be used successfully. You may need to schedule appointments and holidays to take account of this.

Briefing of staff

In the league table of factors contributing to the failure of a clinical study, inadequate briefing of staff comes a close second to deficiency of patients. Investigators grossly underestimate the amount of information they have acquired about the study drug, protocol, methodology and case report form; they also underestimate the time and effort needed to communicate that information to others. Furthermore, most clinicians (like ordinary mortals) are poor teachers.

If you cannot do the entire study yourself, you must do at least the following:

- Supply copies of protocol and case report form to all staff involved.
- Supply (or lend) copies of the Investigators' Brochure to any clinicians who will have responsibility for subjects in the study.
- Hold at least one pre-study meeting (see Chapter 5) to review drug, protocol and case report form. Do not lecture to your audience, unless you have a track record of keeping listeners awake for longer than 5 minutes; make the participants in turn review or summarise the important issues. This ensures that at least one of the group is giving the matter full attention, and encourages the others to listen critically.
- Demonstrate all measurement techniques to be used in the study. More importantly, test the ability of your staff to perform the methods. Do not take anything for granted: you cannot assume that even the blood pressure will be taken in the same way by different individuals. In some cases you may have to do a preliminary study to check inter-observer variability.
- Make sure that all are aware of the need for meticulous record keeping. Nurses are usually well-trained in this respect, but many physicians are resistant to training in such seemingly mundane matters.
- Pay special attention to procedures for handling biological samples. Your assistants may never have separated red cells from plasma or serum, or store a haematology specimen. Furthermore, it is a rule of clinical research that the novice will always discard at least one urine collection after measuring its volume but before saving an aliquot.
- Teach your assistants to treat the study subjects as

royalty, or better.

- Give all staff a list of contact names, telephone numbers and addresses.
- Make sure that the code-breaking procedure is known to all who might need it (see below).
- Specify, preferably in writing, where assistants can find:
  Keys to department, drug storage cupboard, filing cabinet
  Consumables for routine procedures and for specialised equipment
  Help with defective equipment
  New and part-completed case report forms
  Another copy of the study protocol.
- Teach everyone to refer to the study protocol in the event of uncertainty or disagreement.
- Encourage everyone to contact the study sponsor if in doubt about almost anything.

Use of drugs

Supply

Before you schedule a study and recruit any subjects, you must be absolutely certain that the test medication will arrive in time. Most pharmaceutical companies have to complete extensive procedures before they can release any medication to a clinician, and their rules are usually inflexible. For example, they need written confirmation of Ethics Committee approval and in many countries official clearance for importation. Make sure that the sponsor knows when the first treatment is to be given, and be sceptical of quoted delivery dates.

Storage

Think long and hard before deciding to store medication anywhere other than in a hospital pharmacy. Security is poor in many academic departments, and the theft of medication is an embarrassing and dangerous possibility. Pharmacists are likely to obey storage and dispensing instructions to the letter, and will continue to function even if you are ill or on holiday.

Accountability

The sponsor has a permanent responsibility to ensure the safe consumption of study medication, and some form of record of its receipt, dispensing, disposal and return is clearly needed. You should therefore expect to be asked to maintain a written record of amounts used and stock remaining. The layout of the drug accountability form resembles a bank statement, functions in the same way and has the same significance. Using the hospital pharmacy for drug storage and dispensing will relieve you of the simple but unrewarding job of maintaining this record for which, as the investigator, you are ultimately responsible.

Drug administration: procedures for checking and recording

Errors in the administration of medication have greater potential to wreck a study than has almost any other act or omission, particularly in volunteer studies where the total number of subjects is small. For example, giving the wrong treatment in a randomised crossover study may at a stroke invalidate many pages of data, and will certainly unbalance the order of treatments. If the wrong treatment is given to one subject, that error is often matched by a reciprocal error in another subject. In repeated dose studies, a single dose of active drug may invalidate an entire period of treatment with placebo. Omission of the penultimate dose may devalue the pharmacokinetic assessments scheduled to be made after the final dose.

In spite of the seriousness of errors in drug administration, it is hard to maintain the high level of vigilance needed to prevent them.

The following checking procedures should help:

- Put wristband labels on the subjects for the duration of the study. The label can bear the subject's name and number, the study code number, and the clinician's name or telephone number for use in emergencies.
- Always ask the patient's name, even if you think you know it. Use a form of words such as 'Please tell me your name' rather than 'Are you Mrs Jones?', since the answer to the latter question is likely to be 'Yes' even if the patient's name is Williams.
- Check the labelling on the medication against the relevant page in the case record form. Make sure that you have the correct case record form.
- Ask an assistant to check the medication positively rather than negatively. Your helper should check the identity of the subject once agian, and check the trial medication as above. This is helped by both reading the instructions aloud in the presence of the other.
- If the subject says 'That's not the same as the tablet I had yesterday' they are probably right and you should check the whole procedure once more.

These procedures may seem tedious, or even insulting, to the clinician administering the medication. Without such obsessive care, however, mistakes are certain to occur and can be a disaster for everyone.

Safety monitoring

Investigators sometimes view 'safety monitoring' as an unproductive chore. The study sponsor should certainly match the safety tests to the nature and degree of any hazard, since measures that are perceived as unnecessary are likely to be done badly. On the other hand, the clinician should be aware that most potential drugs fail because of unexpected toxicity.

The following safety tests are included in almost every drug study.

Vital signs

It is surely sensible to measure pulse rate and blood pressure in early studies on any potential drug, even if no cardiovascular or autonomic effects are anticipated. Measurements in the standing position are a greater challenge to the subject's homeostatic mechanisms than those done with the subject supine. Respiratory rate and body temperature are less likely to be useful, but are easy to measure. Even if there is no obvious justification for recording vital signs, their inclusion does at least ensure that the subject is regularly observed at close quarters.

Laboratory screening tests

These usually comprise a battery (or, less aggressively, a 'profile') of tests on blood and urine samples. Abnormalities occurring in a single patient are often impossible to interpret, and this devalues the use of the tests, in the eyes of the clinician. However, the real value of these test batteries becomes apparent as soon as data are available from many patients receiving the test drug, and is further enhanced if placebo data are also obtained. Occasionally laboratory screening tests become markedly abnormal in a substantial proportion of treated patients, and this evidence may be enough to halt the development of the drug. For these reasons the untargeted use of laboratory tests in clinical drug studies is fully justified, and any remarkable abnormalities in them should be reported to the sponsor so that they may be reviewed in the light of reports from other centres or studies.

If you have not studied healthy volunteers previously, you may be surprised by the high prevalence of laboratory results that are outside the normal range. There are innocent explanations for some of these, such as the raised transaminases or creatine phophokinase levels seen after severe muscular exercise. Other 'abnormalities' reflect the statistical definition of a 'normal range' as 2 standard deviations either side of the mean. Finally, you should remember that tests performed without any clinical indication cannot be interpreted in the same way as tests that have been done for diagnostic or prognostic purposes.

Recording adverse events

The case report form will contain pages designed for the recording of adverse events (AE) that occur during the study. You will probably find these unsatisfactory because the structure of the form makes it difficult for you to describe all the clinical details comprehensively. Nevertheless, a restrictive structure is needed so that AE can be coded, grouped and analysed when data from many patients are available.

Remember that all AE should be recorded not merely those that you feel might be treatment-related. The relationship between drug and AE can be properly assessed only when substantial experience has been gained with the compound. Many AE report forms ask you to judge the probability that the AE was caused by the drug, but it is rarely possible to do this with confidence.

Handling adverse events

Adverse events in clinical studies need open and sympathetic handling. In view of the difficulty in determining relationship to treatment in individual cases, it is best always to accept that the AE might have been caused by the study drug. Curiously, patients and volunteers are often eager to blame factors outside the study; perhaps that is an alternative to reproaching themselves for, as they might see it, risking their health by participating.

Healthy volunteers who are injured as a result of taking part in a study should be compensated by the sponsor, even if no-one is to blame, as recommended by the Association of the British Pharmaceutical Industry. The amount of compensation is that which might have been awarded by a court had negligence been proved. Happily, studies in normal people have a very good safety record. If important injuries do occur, however, the sponsor must be notified as soon as possible so that the company can take responsibility for the matter. Do not make promises to the subject about compensation, unless the sponsor asks you to do so. Keep your professional defence organisation informed, even if you believe it unlikely that legal action will be taken against you.

If a patient or volunteer is injured in your study, it does no harm to express your regret. A secretive and defensive approach is inappropriate in these circumstances and is probably more likely to lead to legal dispute than is an open and sympathetic attitude.

Reporting adverse events

Reporting of AE is an important component of 'good clinical practice' (see Chapter 11) and is of great concern to pharmaceutical companies. As you would expect, study sponsors invariably require that you report serious AE within 24 hours, not least because your report might have implications for the welfare of other subjects in the study.

However, some aspects of the usual definition of 'serious AE' may at first glance seem unhelpful:

a) Requiring, or prolonging, inpatient hospitalisation
b) Disabling
c) Life-threatening
d) Death
e) Malignancy
f) Congenital anomaly

You may be reluctant to report examples of d, e or f as 'serious' because the circumstances of the AE were such that the study drug was almost certainly not to blame. You must report them nevertheless; the sponsor, the author of the study report, and the regulatory authorities should be more than capable of reaching the same conclusion, so notifying the AE will do no scientific damage. If you are uncertain about whether an AE is 'serious' or otherwise worthy of notification, you should not hesitate to contact the sponsor for discussion and guidance.

Withdrawal of subjects

You will find it painful to withdraw a subject from your study, because of the time and effort you have already invested. However, you must not feel under pressure to continue; the subject's welfare is paramount, and if you are in any doubt whether to continue you should consider asking a disinterested colleague to advise. Data from withdrawn subjects are not wasted. They will be included in the analysis of tolerability and may make a valuable contribution to the safety profile of the drug. Incomplete data may sometimes be useful in the efficacy analysis also.

Withdrawals must be followed up in at least as much detail as the subjects completing the study. Do not discard any of the data or biological samples.

Follow up

Healthy volunteers

It is unusual for a protocol to specify that volunteers be followed up for longer than 1 week after the end of the final treatment period. For that reason, it is important that the family practitioner is informed about the study so that the details will form a permanent part of the medical record. If problems that might be attributable to the study drug were to arise months or years later, the subject's physician should then be able to contact the investigator or sponsor.

Very rarely, a potential drug is found to have severe toxicity only after it has been given to volunteers. In that case, the sponsor has a responsibility to trace the recipients of the compound and to arrange appropriate counselling and surveillance.

Patients

Follow-up of patients in the UK is easier than that of volunteers, because the patients are studied in the context of the National Health Service. However, it remains important to ensure that the family practitioner is fully informed about the patient's participation, since hospital records may be lost, investigators may move to posts elsewhere, or the hospital may be closed. Patients who have received a toxic compound may need tracing and prolonged follow-up, as with healthy volunteers (see above).

The study protocol should include provision for patients to continue on the trial medication if it has suited them well. There would clearly be ethical objections to giving patients an effective treatment and then withdrawing it.

Handling emergencies

When medical emergencies occur during a study, there is a tendency for physicians (other than the investigators) to behave as if paralysed by the knowledge that the patient is receiving an experimental drug. In practice, most serious medical problems arising in a study are unrelated to the trial medication and can usually be treated conventionally. However, specialised knowledge of the study drug may be needed to plan the patient's management correctly, and for that reason it is important make available to patient and family practitioner the contact names and telephone numbers of the investigator and the sponsor. These could be written on the subject's wristband and study subjects should be issued with a card giving information where you or your associates can be reached 24h per day for advice to the subject or his physicians.

Procedures for code breaking In studies of healthy subjects it is rarely necessary to break the treatment code, because knowledge of the treatment does not influence the management of the clinical problem; furthermore, interpretation of the data may be biased once the identity of the treatment is known. In studies of patients, the code has to be broken more often because the identity of the trial medication might influence the management of an intercurrent illness or an exacerbation of pre-existing disease. In all cases, the clinician responsible for the subject must have the power to break the code, and procedures to allow this must be set out in the protocol.

Copies of the treatment code must be held by each investigator and the sponsor independently. It may be sensible for the investigators to keep copies in their homes as well as their hospitals although the security of the codes has to be assured.

The treatment code must be kept in separate envelopes for each subject and study period so that the code can be broken for a single patient and period without revealing any information that is not needed.

In large multi-centre studies, local procedures may be replaced by a single surveillance centre that provides a 24-hour code-breaking facility via the telephone. In a hospital the pharmacy is a good place to manage the emergency decoding.

Study discontinuation If one of your patients experiences a severe adverse event in a drug study, you may lose your appetite for the project and might well decide to stop recruiting further patients. Do not be surprised if the sponsor continues the study in other centres; their decision may be more objective than yours because their view is not coloured by personal contact with the patient.

Rarely, toxicity of a trial drug is such that the entire

study is discontinued. More commonly, a protocol amendment (Chapter 6) is needed to allow a reduction in dose. If a study is stopped because of poor tolerability, you must allow time with the patients for extensive discussion of the problems and their implications.

Protocol compliance versus optimum patient care

The welfare of study subjects must always take precedence over the requirements of the protocol. A well thought-out protocol will not conflict with the interests of the patient; if conflict does arise, the protocol may be amended accordingly. If the sponsor will not agree to a protocol amendment, then you must either deviate from the protocol or withdraw the subject. If the necessary deviation from protocol would invalidate that subject's data, withdrawal is the only possible action.

Monitoring visits

Good Clinical Practice (see Chapter 11) places a clear obligation upon the sponsor to monitor the study regularly with suitably qualified and experienced staff. You must therefore set aside time for these visits, which typically occur about every 6 weeks, dep. The monitor (or Clinical Research Associate/CRA) will need access to source data in order to verify the accuracy and integrity of the case report form, and will probably spend half a day in your unit on each visit. You should allow about 1.5 hours in which to answer queries and supply original records for inspection. You may find that tedious, but it is now essential: the sponsor has to be seen to have monitored the study correctly if the data are to be accepted by governmental regulatory authorities for medicines.

The monitors' job is to ensure the satisfactory completion of the study, and you should regard them as valuable allies. If you need any help, ask for it.

Keeping up the momentum

Some studies never get off the ground, and a few progress rapidly to a successful conclusion. Most studies, however, start well but then stall and stagger because of slow recruitment of subjects. The study monitors are all too familiar with this phenomenon, but can do little to help apart from encouraging, reminding and 'pressurising' you. If recruitment is suffering because of unnecessarily restrictive inclusion/exclusion criteria, ask the sponsor whether the protocol requirements can be relaxed. If that cannot be done, re-examine the suggestions given at the start of this chapter. If you find those unhelpful, do not

despair. Dogged persistence usually wins through in the end.

11

Good clinical practice

Jean Soul-Lawton and Ria Kroon

Introduction

The term Good Clinical Practice (GCP) suggests that it relates to a standard of practical clinical medicine; it does not. It is a standard, or more precisely, a set of standards that have been developed for the conduct of clinical trials with investigative new drugs. These standards can actually be applied to any experimentation in humans. The general aim of Good Clinical Practice is to **protect subjects' rights** and **ensure the accuracy of the data collection** (see Box 11.1).

Good Clinical Practice was first defined in the USA in 1977 as a result of concerns about the quality and authenticity of some of the research data submitted to the regulatory authorities for drug registration. Since then, Good Clinical Practice guidelines have been defined in Europe, the USA and Japan.

In July 1996 The International Conference on Harmonisation (ICH) guideline on Good Clinical Practice was adopted by the CPMP (European Union) followed by MHW (Japan) in March 1997. The FDA (USA) published the ICH/GCP guidelines in the Federal Register in May 1997. The objective of this ICH GCP guideline is to provide a unified standard for the European Union (EU), Japan and the United States to facilitate the mutual acceptance of clinical data by the regulatory authorities in these jurisdictions. The guideline was developed with consideration of the good clinical practices of the European Union, Japan and the United States, as well as those of Australia, Canada, the Nordic countries and the World Health Organisation (WHO).

The contents of this chapter may seem a little intimidating and perhaps they suggest that bureaucracy has won the day. Certainly, there is an element of bureaucracy about GCP, but there is little doubt that implementation of GCP can improve the quality of clinical research as well as demonstrating that the data collected are indeed reliable and authentic. The investigator will need to work with a clinical trial monitor who should not be regarded as someone making personal criticism but rather

Box 11.1 Good clinical practice

A standard by which clinical trials are designed, implemented and reported so that there is public assurance that the data are credible and that the rights, integrity and confidentiality of subjects are protected.

This involves:

- Establishment of procedures for protection of patients:
  - Informed consent
  - Ethics committees
- Establishment of a paper trail for verification of data
- Effective monitoring of the investigator by sponsoring drug companies
- Inspection by authorities to ensure:
  - Adequate systems
  - Accurate records

as an ally, someone who can help you to attain a high standard of clinical research.

Legal status The importance of Good Clinical Practice is such that it has legal status, though this differs markedly between countries. In the USA, a number of regulations define the responsibilities of the investigator, the sponsor (pharmaceutical company), the trial monitor and the Institutional Review Board (IRB)/Ethics Committee. Some of these regulations are enforceable in law and investigators, sponsors and IRBs are all subject to inspection (audit) by the FDA (see below).

In Europe, many countries have now adopted legislation on Good Clinical Practice. The ICH guidelines have been adopted by the CPMP since July 1996. At present, the guidelines are used by the pharmaceutical industry and it is expected that all company and external personnel involved with the setting up and running of a clinical trial will adhere to this standard. Anyone involved in clinical drug research will at some time be exposed to these regulations. A European Directive on Clinical Trials is under development. The purpose of this European Directive is to accelerate and ease the preparation and execution of international multi-centre trials in Europe without affecting the accuracy of data collection or the protection of the subjects' rights. All EU countries will have to adapt their legal systems to this directive when it is accepted.

Box 11.2 Responsibilities of the investigator

- To supply credentials (e.g. provision of curriculum vitae)
- To familiarise himself with the properties of the investigational drug
- To ensure confidentiality of information
- To provide adequate resources and time to conduct the clinical trial
- To inform staff involved
- To ensure that recruitment rate of patients is sufficient
- To reach agreement with the sponsor regarding the protocol, Good Clinical Practice, monitoring procedures and publication of data
- To submit the protocol to an ethics committee
- To obtain informed consent from the study subjects
- If appropriate, inform subject's GP.
- To establish a system for drug storage, handling, accountability, randomisation and blinding
- To ensure proper collection and handling of data
- To report adverse events and assure patient safety
- If appropriate, to submit summaries of trial status to the ethical committee annually.
- To agree to data validation, source document verification and audit
- To provide a report of the trial
- To assure retention of trial documentation/patient records
- To take medical responsibility for the study subjects and provision of emergency resuscitation equipment

How can GCP be achieved?

For an individual study, procedures are controlled by what is written in the protocol, and the case report form (CRF). In addition, Standard Operating Procedures (SOPs) are used to describe general processes which can be applied to many studies. Pharmaceutical companies instigate regular monitoring of the study and continually gather together documentation which should be adequate to withstand audit where it will be checked if the SOPs were correctly followed. Investigators must also write SOPs to establish and maintain the standard of conduct of studies within their unit.

SOPs

Standard Operating Procedures are instruction manuals written for carrying out a study from start to finish. SOPs often specify details which are not given in the protocol and include, for example, detailed procedures for calibrating or operating specialised equipment. In order to comply with EC Good Clinical Practice guidelines, pharmaceutical companies should have SOPs for conducting all of their clinical studies. The SOPs should be written so that relatively inexperienced or new staff can establish exactly what needs to be done. Once written, SOPs need to be checked periodically and amended when procedures change.

The investigator

Clearly, the investigator is a key person in the trial. The responsibilities of the investigator defined in the ICH/GCP guidelines are summarised in Box 11.2.

All of these issues need to be considered before the study starts. In the USA, an integral part of the IND (Investigational New Drug) application is a 'Statement of Investigator' which has to be completed by each investigator involved in the studies (Forms FD1572 and FD1573). Completion of these forms by investigators in Europe is required if studies are being carried out under an IND. These forms ask for the investigator's education and experience and details of any clinical laboratory facilities which will be used. They also ask for assurance that an institutional review board (ethics committee) will be involved in the study and that the drug will be used under the supervision of the investigator in accordance with the protocol.

Clinical trial monitoring

Monitoring of a clinical trial is a key element of Good Clinical Practice and is a method of providing quality control (see below). Even in the most organised of clinical trial centres, simple errors can be made, for example, in transcribing data from a patient's notes to a CRF. The clinical trial monitor's role starts before the trial begins and continues after the last subject has completed the study. For a pharmaceutical company-sponsored trial, the clinical trial monitor, whose responsibilities are defined in the ICH/GCP guidelines, forms an essential link with the investigator (see Box 11.3). The investigator can expect that the monitor is adequately qualified to ensure knowledgeable supervision of the trial. When the study is up and running the monitor may make many visits to check that the trial is being carried out according to the protocol and that data are being collected and recorded properly. The monitor will interact with the investigator at different stages of the study.

Pre-study visit At this visit the monitor will discuss the feasibility of carrying out the study at the investigator site, and is likely

Box 11.3 Responsibilities of the monitor

- To work according to predetermined standard operating procedures
- To visit the investigator before during and after the trial to ensure:
  - Adherence to the protocol
  - Complete and accurate data collection
  - Informed consent is obtained and recorded
- To ensure that facilities in the trial site including laboratories staff and equipment are adequate
- To ensure that recruitment rate of subjects will be adequate
- To ensure that staff assisting the investigator has been informed about the details of the trial
- To ensure communication between investigator and sponsor
- To check entries in case report forms against the source documents
- To check storage and dispensing of study drugs
- To assist the investigator with notification to authorities and with reporting the results to the sponsor
- To keep records of all visits or other contacts with the investigator (monitoring reports)

to cover the following issues:

- Investigator's brochure
  This should be supplied by the company in order to provide relevant background information about the study drug (see Chapter 3). The investigator's brochure, along with the protocol is a confidential document and the monitor may ask for a confidentiality document to be signed.

- Protocol
  This needs to be signed by the investigator.

- Recruitment
  The monitor should be assured that there is a good possibility that the required number of subjects can be recruited in the desired time frame. Data on the number of potentially eligible subjects seen in the preceding months at the investigator site may be requested.

- Resources
  Adequate staff and resources (personnel, equipment, laboratory facilities) should be available throughout the study.

- Handling of samples
  Procedures must be established for the collection of samples (blood, urine, etc) and for these to be kept under the correct storage conditions before analysis. It may be necessary for the company to supply the appropriate collection tubes, labels and forms, etc.

- Drug storage
  In most cases drug (with randomisation code, if appropriate) is stored in the pharmacy at the investigator site and dispensed to the investigator as required. The investigator is responsible for keeping track of the drug and ensuring storage conditions are appropriate and that the drug is dispensed in accordance with the protocol. The investigator is also responsible for accounting for all drug and returning unused drug.

- Confidentiality
  All personnel involved in carrying out the study should be aware of the need to maintain confidentiality of information regarding subjects entered into the trial.

- Informed consent
  The information sheet for the subjects and the informed consent procedure will be discussed.

- Ethics Committee
  It is the responsibility of the investigator to seek Ethics Committee approval. The protocol and consent form will have to be reviewed and approved by the local Ethics Committee and a letter stating this should be provided and filed.

- Documentation
  Reading through the CRF will give an idea of the paperwork involved for each subject entered into the trial. Other documentation will be discussed.

- Monitoring
  A clear line of communication must be established and maintained between the monitor and the investigator. The frequency of monitoring procedures and the carrying out of source document verification should be discussed and agreed.

- Source document verification
  This is an essential part of the monitoring procedure. Source documents are those where the data were recorded first, e.g. patient notes, original clinical/physiological recordings. The FDA is reluctant to accept data generated without proper document verification, and the ICH Good Clinical Practice guidelines state that it is the investigator's responsibility to make data available for this. There are obvious implications for patient confidentiality which must be taken into account and local regulations/codes must be upheld.

- Good Clinical Practice
  The investigator and co-investigators must provide a curriculum vitae, and the normal ranges from the laboratory being used at the site must be supplied. The investigator should confirm that he understands and will comply with Good Clinical Practice procedures, and it should be understood that a data trail needs to be established.

- Report and publications
  Provisions for analysis of the data, the study report and publications should be discussed and agreed.

- Payment
  Finances required for the study may include an honorarium for the investigator, payment of volunteers, expenses of trial subjects, payment for tests etc., and have to be calculated and agreed. The details of finances provided may be requested by, for example, the health authority, via the Ethics Committee.

- Liability/compensation
  Insurance against injury to the subjects taking part in the trial should be clarified by the monitor and will usually be stated in the protocol. The liability of the

investigator and sponsor should also be clarified.

Initiation visit Having agreed the feasibility of carrying out the trial with the investigator, the monitor will return to discuss the study again with the investigator and all the other personnel involved, e.g. other medical staff, clinical research nurses. The pharmacist should also be involved in discussions. He may be responsible for administration of the drug according to a randomisation code and should be fully aware of the investigator, protocol, drug formulation, quantity, delivery dates, storage conditions and length and time of the study. For a blinded trial, a system must be agreed for providing access to the randomisation code for individual subjects in case of an emergency, for example, a serious adverse event.

Before the study can start, the monitor needs to ensure that the study drug has arrived, that the investigator has all the CRFs and that Ethics Committee approval has been obtained in writing.

Trial file The monitor is likely to request the setting up of a trial file by the investigator (already discussed in Chapter 5). This should contain all the documentation (e.g. Ethics Committee approval, all correspondence between the company and the investigator) regarding the study to satisfy audit. There are also guidelines that state in considerable detail which documents should be available at the investigator site and the monitor will check that these are available.

Monitoring visit The first visit will often be after entry of only two or three subjects to ensure that the protocol is being adhered to and that the investigator has not, for example, misunderstood entry criteria. If new staff join the study the monitor will need to know for contacting purposes and to ensure that they are adequately briefed. The monitor will discuss problems in recruitment if the rate is slower than expected and will check the following:

- Informed consent forms
- The investigator's trial file
- Storage and dispensing of drug

- Completion and legibillty of CRFs and accuracy of the data are accurate when compared with source documents.

  Complete, accurate and legible forms will be critical for data analysis and adherence to Good Clinical Practice. Photocopies of CRFs are often needed and for this reason they are best completed in black ink. When an error in entry is made the incorrect entry should be crossed out once and the correct entry added, dated and signed by the investigator.

  The subject should be identifiable by a number only. The subject may also be identified by initials, but not their full name in order to maintain confidentiality. The subject number will usually be the means of identifying a subject once he is entered and will appear on every page of the CRF to ensure that if a page of the CRF is separated from the rest it can be related to a specific subject.

- Correct reporting of adverse events

- Protocol violations and non-compliance with the protocol.

- Status of randomisation code

  Breaking the randomisation code for an individual subject during a study should only be carried out when absolutely necessary to avoid bias. For example, when a serious adverse event has occurred information on the drug administered may be needed in order to take the appropriate action. Justification for breaking the code should be given in the CRF and the monitor should be informed.

- Study termination

  Specific information on whether a subject completed a trial or not will often be requested on CRFs as the FDA requires annual IND reports giving details of the patient population exposed to a study drug in clinical trials worldwide. To satisfy this, details are required of normal completion, premature discontinuation and death.

- Protocol violations

  Non-compliance with the protocol will be recorded and

should be pointed out to the investigator

- Adverse events

An adverse event/experience is defined in the ICH/GCP guidelines as 'any untoward occurrence in a patient or clinical investigation subject administered a pharmaceutical product and which does not necessarily have a causal relationship with this treatment'.

A serious adverse event is defined as one that is fatal, life-threatening, disabling or that requires hospitalisation or prolongs pre-existing hospitalisation. Congenital abnormality and cancer are always to be regarded as serious. The FDA include overdose with this definition. The investigator should also be aware of and report unexpected adverse experiences; that is, an adverse experience not previously reported in nature, severity and incidence in the Investigator's Brochure or elsewhere.

It is stated in the ICH/GCP guidelines that it is the investigator's responsibility to notify (with documentation) the sponsor (pharmaceutical company) and when applicable, ethics committee and relevant authorities immediately in the case of a serious adverse event and to take appropriate measures to safeguard subjects. The FDA guidelines require serious adverse events to be reported by telephone within 3 working days; many pharmaceutical companies usually request that serious adverse events are reported by telephone within 24 hours of the event. This should be followed by a hard copy of the serious adverse event form as soon as possible, but at least within ten working days. The company has a responsibility to analyse the serious adverse event pattern as soon as possible as it may be necessary to alter the protocol or adjust dosage or safety monitoring procedures.

- Sign-off

GCP requires that the investigator sign the CRFs that are returned to the pharmaceutical company; however, signing the CRFs is not a requirement of the FDA.

The site monitoring visit is an essential part of the monitor's job. Both the FDA and ICH/GCP guidelines require frequent monitoring visits to sites where clinical studies are being carried out. The frequency of visits depends on the duration of the study and the number of subjects involved. Short studies (1-2 months or less) where subjects are recruited quickly may need to be visited frequently whereas longer term studies (3m-1y+) are likely to be visited less frequently, that is approximately every four weeks.

Close down visit

The monitor will need to ensure that the CRFs are complete and that the investigator has a copy of all of them. The monitor will remove any unused or returned drug (or it can be destroyed locally under the appropriate conditions), study materials and equipment provided by the company. All drug should be accounted for and envelopes containing the code for a double blind study should be given to the monitor. The monitor will leave all informed consent forms and the drug log (having taken a copy of the drug log) with the investigator.

The monitor will still have responsibilities even though the centre is closed for recruitment. Data queries may need resolving regarding subjects entered into the study. The principal investigator will have to agree and sign the final report and must be aware that the site could be subject to audit.

Archiving

Once the clinical trial is completed, it is necessary for the investigator to archive clinical trial documentation which can be made available for audit. Patient files and other source data must be kept for the maximum period of time permitted by the hospital, institution or private practice, but not less than 2 years after the last approval of a marketing application in an ICH region and until there are no pending or contemplated marketing applications in an ICH region or at least 2 years have elapsed since the formal discontinuation of the clinical development of the investigational product (ICH/GCP guidelines).

Quality control and quality assurance

The ICH/GCP guidelines define quality assurance (QA) as 'all those planned and systematic actions that are established to ensure that the trial is performed and the data are generated (documented) and reported in compliance with Good Clinical Practice and the applicable regulatory requirements(s). This is validated through in-process quality and in- and post-process auditing, both being applied to the clinical trial process as well as to the data. In practice, this means that companies should have good SOPs for all the procedures involved in a clinical trial, and in addition should audit their investigators.

The guidelines define quality control (QC) as 'operational techniques and activities undertaken within the system of quality assurance to verify that the requirements for quality of the trial have been fulfilled'. QC activities concern all members of the investigational team including the staff of the sponsor involved with planning, conducting, monitoring, evaluating and reporting a trial including data processing, with the objective of avoiding trial subjects being exposed to unnecessary risks, or false conclusions being drawn from unreliable data.

Monitoring is the most important means of carrying out QC activities in the process of setting up and running a clinical trial and has already been described. If QC procedures discover deficiencies, for example, that data are inadequate in the CRF, steps must be taken to prevent the problem recurring and it must be decided whether inadequate data can be amended or cannot be used at all. Clearly, discovering deficiencies early on is crucial. QC activities are carried out by personnel responsible for the study because they must be aware of how well the study procedures are operating.

For the purposes of quality assurance, QC procedures should be documented so that it can be verified that they were carried out regularly and that where necessary, remedial action was taken.

Audit and inspection

The FDA routinely audits investigator sites for compliance with Good Clinical Practice, and this includes sites in Europe which have provided data for drug registration in the USA. As Good Clinical Practice is incorporated in the pharmaceutical laws of European countries their authorities will also undertake audits of investigators.

The routine inspection of clinical investigators carried out by the FDA is generally divided into two parts. One part deals with the practical side of the study, for example, which personnel carried out particular trial activities, where precisely the study took place and when and how the drug was stored. The interaction between the monitor and investigator are also assessed, and documentation relating to monitoring visits should be available in the investigator's records, as should correspondence with the ethics committee. The second part of the inspection involves audit of the data itself. The data submitted to the FDA will be compared against records kept at the investigator site from which the data may be derived. These include, for example, hospital notes to examine a patient's history and ensure that the subject fitted study entry criteria according to the protocol. Measurements taken during the course of the study and any laboratory results may be inspected, and records may be checked to ensure that side-effects were reported appropriately. A copy of the signed consent form should be kept in each trial subject's records. The FDA audit usually involves a detailed check of a few selected subjects. The audit may include the (bio)chemical analytical facilities at the site if applicable.

Further reading

- EC (1990). Good Clinical Practice for Trials on Medicinal Products in the European Community. III/3976/88-EN Final [Approved July 1990; effective July 1991]. Published in: Pharmacology and Toxicology 67: 361-72.
- ICH Harmonised Tripartite Guideline, E6 Guideline for Good Clinical Practice, Step 5, 1.7.1996 (CPMP/ICH/135/95).

Useful Websites for finding full text of guidelines

- International Conference on Harmonisation (ICH) http://www.pharmweb.net/pwmirror/pw9/ifpma/ich1.html

- FDA Guidance pages;
  http://www.fda.gov/cder/guidance/index.htm
  On this website you can access all documents on drug development issued by the US Food and Drug Administration.
- The European Agency for the Evaluation of Medicinal Products;http://www.eudra.org/en_home.htm
  This website provides access to the full text of all regulatory guidelines in addition to other useful guidelines issued by the European Medicines Agency. This includes the ICH documents - which can also be found on the FDA site.

12

Communicating Clinical Research

Peter van Brummelen, Douglas E. Busch and Karin le Poole

Introduction

Communication is essential for the progress of science. Only after you have documented your work in such a way that other scientists can analyse it and build on it, is your study complete. Communication has also become important for career development, and every research worker looking for promotion is expected to present a record of successful communications.

Ideally, you should aim to publish your work as an original paper in a peer-reviewed scientific journal. A written document has the advantage that it provides a permanent, detailed record which can be disseminated widely. Publication in an established journal adds credibility, because of the selection and publishing processes involved. A quicker way to communicate your findings is by oral presentations or posters at meetings.These methods allow a more direct interaction with your target audience and help you to develop ideas for the final publication, but cannot replace it. Even if they are later published in a conference proceedings, effective oral presentations and posters do not contain the same detail as an original paper written for publication.

Before starting to prepare any sort of scientific communication, it is important to find out if there are any limitations to the amount of information you may disclose. Would communication infringe any secrecy agreements or invalidate a patent application at a later date? Also, has the work already been published or submitted for publication elsewhere? With a few exceptions (publication in different languages or for different audiences), duplicate or repeat publication is considered unethical and should be avoided.

Writing for publication

Research is considered to be worth publishing when it extends existing knowledge or its practical applications. Check that your findings fulfil one of these criteria before starting to write. Also confirm that the study was properly designed (see Chapter 7) and conducted according to the approved protocol (see Chapters 6 and 10), that all the data have been recorded accurately and the statistical methods used are valid (see Chapter 8). Do your conclusions answer the question you set out to study?

If you are satisfied with the answers you get, aim to produce a full report of high quality. Publication before the termination of a long-term study may be considered if preliminary findings show a definite trend and could influence future research. In such a case, a short report or 'letter to the editor' is more appropriate. However, do not be tempted to split a study into several papers ('salami science') unless you have good reason for it. Many studies performed for pharmaceutical companies will initially be written up as a very detailed study report (Chapter 13) which may serve as the basis for a subsequent scientific publication.

Selecting a journal

At an early stage you should choose your target journal and write specifically for that particular journal. Your choice depends on several factors:

- Who are you writing for (e.g. scientists in general, medical practitioners, medical specialists, other workers in your field)?
- Do your findings have global significance or are they limited to a particular geographic area?
- Which language are you planning to write in?
- Which journals publish the type of paper you are proposing to write?
- Which of these journals have a good scientific reputation?
- Which journals process and publish papers quickly?
- Which journals are available on Internet and are they to be found in full text or with only their contents pages and/or abstracts ?
- Which journals are covered by the main indexing and abstracting services (e.g. Index Medicus/Medline, Excerpta Medica)?
- Which journals accept one of the standard methods of citing references (Vancouver or Harvard: see below)?

Do not expect one of the leading international journals to accept your paper unless your findings are close to being a major breakthrough in the field or on a topic that is currently under debate. Such journals often reject up to 90% of papers submitted to them! Also, if a journal has recently published a major study on the same subject as yours, your chances of getting into one of the next editions is reduced.

It can take from a few weeks to over a year for your paper to appear in print after it has been accepted. Journals with a higher publication frequency (weekly or monthly) usually have a shorter delay than quarterly journals. If a journal shows acceptance dates, you can easily calculate the lag. You can also keep delays to a minimum by closely following the journal's instructions to authors.

If photographs in high quality or colour are an important aspect of your paper, be aware that not all journals can print them; those that do may ask you to cover the extra cost. Some journals also have page charges for handling and printing manuscripts or demand payment for reprints.

Basic requirements

Once you have short-listed the most likely candidates, one of the next steps is to look at some recent issues of the chosen journals or their internet website and read their 'Instructions to Authors'. This should give you a better idea about the suitability of each journal for your paper and show you how to proceed further. By following the instructions, you increase the chances that your paper will be accepted, speed up the publishing process and reduce the risk of errors during editing and typesetting.

Many biomedical journals now accept manuscripts prepared in the 'Vancouver style', so-called because it was developed at a meeting of journal editors in Vancouver, Canada in 1978.These 'Uniform requirements for manuscripts submitted to biomedical journals' are designed to make things easier for authors, because you don't need to rewrite the whole paper each time you submit it to a different journal. The latest version of these requirements was published in the JAMA 1997; 277 (11):927-934. Even though a journal claims to accept manuscripts prepared in the Vancouver style, however, you still need to read the journal's own instructions for information about the types of paper accepted, length, languages, number of copies and so on.

It is a good idea at this stage to check that you can supply any additional documents requested (proof of compliance with ethical requirements, copies of informed consent forms, permission from copyright holders to use previously published material, permission to use photos of identifiable persons, statements of financial or other relationships that might lead to a conflict of interests, etc.).

Authorship If you worked in a team rather than alone, you will need to decide before starting to write who will be named as an author and which order names will appear. An author is someone who has contributed significantly to all of the following:

- Conception and design of the study or analysis and interpretation of data, or both
- Drafting the article or revising it for critically important content
- Final approval of the version to be published

Names should be listed according to the importance of each person's contribution. Be sure that everyone agrees, because names after the third place may not appear in reference lists. One person should agree to organise the work and correspond with editors. Check that the name, qualifications and place of work of each author are written correctly.

People who have made a contribution that does not justify their inclusion as authors may be given acknowledgement at an appropriate place in the paper, usually at the end. Such people include supervisors, department heads and other senior colleagues who gave advice, comments or permission for the study, people who helped to collect data or acquire funding, secretaries, nurses and technicians who provided support above their routine duties. Such persons must give their permission to be named.

Manuscript preparation At this point you should be ready to start writing. Write simply and clearly. Remember that your aim is to communicate facts, not to produce a literary masterpiece. Help readers to follow your argumentation by keeping to a recognized structure, by keeping sentences short and straightforward, and by eliminating any information that distracts from your message. Use the active voice (e.g. 'We treated 100 patients', not '100 patients were treated'). The conventional structure for clinical papers is known as IMRAD (Introduction, Methods, Results and Discussion).

The introduction tells the reader why you chose to do this research. It briefly covers the present state of knowledge on the subject (but only what is immediately relevant, not a historical overview), defines which gap in this knowledge your research is designed to fill, and states what you planned to do.

The methods section shows exactly what you did: how you selected and treated patients and controls, how you measured changes, how you analysed the results and established statistical significance, etc. Here you should include enough detail to allow other interested scientists to assess the validity of your results and, if necessary, to repeat the work themselves. All too often, published studies cannot be evaluated, because study design and statistical methodology have been reported too superficially. If the technique you used has already been published in detail, reference to the original paper is sufficient.

The results section states what happened, but without any interpretation. Journals seldom allow enough space to show all the raw data, so processed data are usually acceptable. However, you may supply details on a separate sheet for the journal's reviewers if you wish. Individual findings that differ markedly from the rest, and so might influence the conclusions reached, should be described in detail.

In the discussion section, you can then say what your results mean. How do they fit in with existing knowledge? Do they confirm or contradict previous work? Do they create a need for further studies? Be careful not to condemn other researchers whose work does not fit into your scheme, nor to draw generalised conclusions from a study involving a limited population.

There is no secret formula for successful writing; you will have to find out your own preferred method. Some people write down everything as it comes to mind, organising and deleting later. One way to do this is to write each piece of information on a separate card and then rearrange the order until everything seems to be in the right place. If you are writing in a team, the best way to avoid omissions and repetitions by the individual writers is to start off with an outline. This can be an organised list of topics or short sentences showing the key statements. Whichever way you choose to write, expect to have to prepare several drafts before typing the final manuscript.

The title The title of your paper is the part that will be read most often: in the list of contents of the journal that publishes it; in secondary services such as Current Contents, in computerised databases that may be accessed on the internet and, if you are fortunate, in the list of references of other papers. You must therefore be particularly careful that your title accurately describes the contents and attracts the right people to read the paper. A good title is short (not more than 10-12 words) and specific. Avoid trivial words and phrases (e.g. 'a study of'), abbreviations and trade names. On the internet most of the different search engines will search all title words but display the hits in a format where long titles are abbreviated.

Tables and figures Use tables and figures (photographs, drawings, charts and graphs) only when data cannot be expressed clearly in the text. Overuse reduces legibility and increases printing costs. Each table or figure must have clear labels and appropriate legends or footnotes, so as to be independently understandable; it should not repeat information already in the text or in another table or figure. If any of your tables or figures have been published before, you should obtain written consent to use them again from the copyright holder (usually the publisher) and the author.

Design the layout to fit within the text area on the printed page of your target journal. If the page has two or three columns, you can make the layout fit single or multiple column widths. Tables will be typeset by the journal, but you must supply figures in a ready-to-print form. Remember that figures will probably be reduced in size when published, so allow for this and ensure that lines, patterns and lettering will remain clear on reduction. Prepare each table and figure on a separate sheet of paper; number tables and figures independently and indicate their place in the text.

Tables are best for detailed numeric data and for background information on patients. Keep the structure as simple as possible and arrange data so that readers can extract the key information easily. If you group data (e.g. patients according to age) take care that grouping is correct (e.g. with age grouping '40 to 45' and '45 to 50' those aged 45 can be in both groups; with age grouping 'under 45' and 'over 45' those aged 45 are in neither group). Give units of measure in the headings, not in the body of the table, choosing suitable units to avoid surplus zeros. Report actual numbers rather than percentages, or show both. However, do not calculate percentages for small numbers (to describe 1 patient in 24 as '4.2% of the patients', for example, is inadmissible). Differentiate clearly between missing data and zero readings.

Charts and graphs show trends and relationships. Choose the most appropriate type for your purpose: scattergraphs for relationships between variables, histograms for frequency distributions, line graphs for continuous changes over time and for trends, vertical bar charts for comparisons over time, horizontal bar charts for comparisons at a specific time, maps for relationships in space, diagrams for relationships in structure, size, etc., algorithms for complicated procedures. To ensure clarity, avoid combining charts, especially when this would mean using different axis values. Produce three-dimensional charts only when really necessary; pseudo-3D may look attractive, but is usually misleading. Make drawings about twice the size you want them to appear in print with lines on the chart thicker than those used for the axes. Use symbols and hatching (patterns) that remain distinct after size reduction. Axes should be labelled with units and values, and should always start at zero unless using a logarithmic scale. Check with your target journal whether you should draw grids or put each drawing in a box (most journals do not) and if you should send the original artwork or a photograph. Any text or numbers that you want to have typeset should be written on an overlay or on a copy, not on the original. To allow reviewers to check the validity of any illustrations, supply the numerical data on which they are based. Be careful with tables and figures on Internet. Quite often special software is needed to view them so this software should be mentioned.

Photographs for publication need to be in sharp focus and rich in contrast. Many journals prefer glossy, black-and-white prints to transparencies. Never send X-ray films or negatives. Modify photos of people so they cannot be identified or, even better, obtain written consent for publication. If size is critical, indicate the magnification used or include a scale in the photo. Show which is the top of the photo if it is not clear. Never write directly on photos; put arrows and lettering on an overlay or on a copy; write identifying text on a label and stick it on the back. Do not mount photos on paper or card and do not attach anything with paper clips or staples.

The abstract

An abstract is an abbreviated, accurate representation of the contents without added information or interpretation. There are two main types: informative and indicative or descriptive. Informative abstracts repeat the key messages of the paper and answer the same questions: Why did you start? What did you do? What did you find? What does it mean? This is the type most commonly required for clinical papers. Indicative abstracts give a general idea of the contents of a paper, but do not contain specific details of methods or results. This type of abstract is usually found in review articles and book chapters. The abstract must be understandable independent of the text, but does not need to repeat information found in the title, as they usually appear together.

Traditionally, the informative abstract was a single paragraph about 150 words long, written in the past tense in complete sentences that follow each other logically. It contained no tables, figures or citations. Nowadays clinical journals generally ask for 'structured abstracts'. These are longer (250 words), have a standardised format and a partly controlled vocabulary. Their purpose is to facilitate peer review, help readers to select appropriate papers more quickly, and allow more precise computerised literature searches.

Guidelines for preparing structured abstracts can be found in the journals' instructions to authors. In most cases, you will be asked to provide the following information:

- *Objective*: Precisely what your study aimed to achieve
- *Design*: The type of study and its duration
- *Setting*: The clinical circumstances under which the study was conducted
- *Participants*: The numbers and characteristics of participants and how they were selected; numbers withdrawn because of side effects
- *Interventions*: The essential features of treatment and other interventions
- *Key outcome measures*: The measurements used to assess participants
- *Results*: The main results found
- *Conclusions*: How you interpreted the results

These headings should be included in the abstract. Most of the information can be given in a telegraphic style. This facilitates literature searches and allows more information to be conveyed in the space available.

Key words

Some journals ask you to supply 3 to 10 key words or phrases to assist indexers to catalogue your paper. Choose terms that characterised your study as closely as possible and put them in the place required (e.g. after the title or the abstract). Usually, you should use established terms such as those from the medical subject headings (MeSH) list used in Index Medicus.

References

References provide additional evidence to support your hypothesis. The sources you cite should therefore be relevant and must be cited accurately. The value of your arguments does not depend on the number of references listed; quality and validity are more important. Whenever possible, verify your references by reading the original paper; quoting from a secondary source always carries the risk that the intermediate author misunderstood or misquoted what was written. This also applies to abstracting services. If you cannot obtain the original paper or if it is in a language you do not understand, it is better to refer to the actual source you used, mentioning that it is a secondary source (e.g. Schwarz 1988, cited by White 1991).

Unpublished work, such as papers submitted to, but not yet accepted by a journal, documents not publicly available (e.g. internal reports), lectures, conference abstracts and personal communications, should not be used as references. You may cite such work in the text, however, provided that you have obtained permission from the copyright holder to do so.

The main problem with references is that there is no uniform style for citing or listing them. The two most widely used are the name-and-year (Harvard) and the sequential-numeric (e.g. Vancouver) styles. In the Harvard style, the authors' last names and the year of publication are shown in parentheses at the appropriate place in the text, and the reference list is arranged alphabetically by the first author's name. If there is more than one reference to the same author for the same year, they are differentiated by adding a, b, etc. after the date (e.g. Smith 1988a, Smith 1988b). In the sequential-numeric system, references are numbered in the order they appear in the text and only the number is shown at the appropriate place. The Vancouver style uses such a sequential-numeric system.

To avoid delays, it is essential to follow the style described in the journal's instructions to authors. However, many journals that accept papers in the Vancouver style may, in fact, publish something different. In this case, you may still follow the guidelines set out in the 'Uniform requirements for manuscripts'. In the Vancouver style, references are numbered according to when they are first mentioned in the text, and are identified by arabic numerals in parentheses. References in tables and figures should be numbered according to where the table or figure is identified in the text. Titles of journals are abbreviated after the style used in Index Medicus. Consult the January issue for a complete list of the journals reviewed. List all authors when there are six or less; if there are more than six, list the first three and add 'et al.'. Do not use full stops after authors' initials or after abbreviated journal names.

The second major problem with references is making sure that all the citations in the text are listed correctly, and that all the references listed have a number at the appropriate place in the text. It might help if you use the Harvard style while preparing your drafts, and only change to the Vancouver style for the final manuscript. Nevertheless, be ready to cross-check again after any revisions that require text to be moved, added or deleted.

Submitting to a journal

When the preliminary manuscripts have been discussed with all the authors, a critical colleague and, perhaps, the head of the department, when you have made all the necessary revisions, when the text has been typed and tables and figures prepared as required by the instructions to authors, and when you have checked the references carefully, your manuscript is ready to send to a journal. Prepare the appropriate number of copies plus at least one set for yourself.

Write a short covering letter to the editor of the chosen journal requesting that your paper be accepted for publication. It should include the title of the paper, the names of the authors, a statement that all of them have read and approved the paper, the address, telephone and fax number of the author responsible for communicating between the editorial office and the other authors, and any other information that might be helpful, such as the type of contribution your paper represents, whether you are willing to meet the cost of colour illustrations, whether the paper has been presented or submitted elsewhere, etc.

Enclose copies of permissions to use published material, to use sensitive personal information of identifiable persons, or to name persons for their contributions. If you used a word processor to prepare the text, and the journal accepts electronic manuscripts, you may enclose your disk in one of the accepted formats in addition to the typed copies now or wait until the paper has been accepted. Put everything in a strong envelope large enough to hold the pages without folding them; protect illustrations with stiff card to prevent damage in the post. If the journal is in a different country, attach a label for the customs, stating: 'scientific manuscript, no commercial value'.

Normally, the editor will immediately confirm receipt of your manuscript and tell you how long it will take to reach a decision. This should be within one to two months. If you do not get an answer after this time, you may write to ask the reason for the delay. The editor has four possible alternatives: to accept your paper in the form submitted, to accept it after modification, to offer to reconsider it after modification, or to reject it.

If your paper is rejected, keep calm. Read the editor's letter to find out the reason before deciding on your next move. Some of the reasons given, and possible actions, are:

- *Your paper is outside the scope of the journal.*
  Send it to another journal.
- *We can only accept a small percentage of papers submitted.*
  You may need to make some improvements before sending it to another journal.
- *The article is too long and needs changes.*
  Make the changes if you feel they are justified, and send it to another journal.
- *The paper contains serious flaws or the evidence is incomplete.*
  If the criticism is justified, make the changes to the best of your ability and send it to another journal. If you are convinced that the editor has made a mistake, write

and explain politely why you think the paper should be reconsidered.

If the editor is ready to accept the paper after you have made certain changes, and you and your co-authors agree that the changes do improve the paper, revise as requested. If you reject any of the suggestions, explain why. It may be necessary to retype pages with major changes. If the editor only offers to 'reconsider' your paper after revision, decide whether the effort is worthwhile. The editor of another journal might think differently.

When your paper is accepted, you will probably be asked to sign over copyright to the journal ('Consent to publish form' and whether you want to order reprints. Depending on how the journal is produced (traditional typesetting, by computer or directly from your manuscript) you will receive one or more proofs for correction. Do this quickly and conscientiously. All you need to do is check that nothing has been left out and that the meaning has not been changed in the process of preparing the paper for publication.

At this stage, never be tempted to rewrite or add material. If the editorial staff have made changes in style or spelling, never revert to your original formulation unless it has altered the meaning. The changes were probably made to conform to the journal's house style or to make the meaning clearer. The sooner you return the proofs, and the fewer corrections are needed, the sooner your paper will appear in print. All the points are summarised in Box 12.1.

Box 12.1 Checklist: Writing for a scientific journal

Study assessment	√
Permission to publish	√
Journal selection	√
Instructions to authors	√
Authorship	√
Outline	√
Title	√
Tables and figure	√
1st draft	√
1st draft discussed and modified	√
Abstract	√
References	√
Critical appraisal	√
Revision	√
Manuscript typed	√
Manuscript checked	√
Covering letter	√
Copies/enclosures	√

Oral presentations

When you wish to speak about your research, do not be tempted to read a text prepared for publication; the criteria for effective oral communication are completely different. A speech has to be shorter and simpler, partly because of the limited time available, but also because listeners cannot remember more than three or four of the points presented; even less if the presentation is poorly structured and complex! Listeners have to follow a presentation at the speed set by the speaker. Unlike readers, they cannot repeat parts that are unclear or study complicated tables and figures at length. Nor can they miss out passages that do not interest them. A speaker also needs to master additional skills. A monotone voice or unclear diction, for example, can easily cause listeners to lose interest or even leave the auditorium.

What to say

Which information you will include in your presentation depends on what you want to achieve, who is in your audience, and the time at your disposal. If you want to convince medical practitioners that the new drug you tested is superior to another, you will need a different approach than if you want to get support from a company for further research or if you want to encourage debate among colleagues. It also makes a difference whether your findings are in line with current thinking or whether you can expect strong opposition from the audience. And it is obvious that you can say more in 30 minutes than in 10.

Formulate 3 to 4 statements that lead the audience towards your objective, list the evidence in support of each argument, and prepare a conclusion emphasizing each point made. When selecting, try to imagine which information will interest your audience most. Use simple language and clarify abstract ideas with concrete examples. Next put the individual sections into a logical sequence and link them together with clear transitions (e.g., After these impressive results, you will surely be interested to learn about the incidence of side effects). This forms the main body of your presentation.

Presentation structure

It would be a mistake, however, to present this information alone. If you start off with an important message that nobody is expecting, you risk that it will either be misunderstood or missed altogether. A good presentation has a clear structure with a distinct beginning, middle and end; the main body of information belongs in the middle.

In the opening phase, you should gain the audience's attention by stating clearly what you are going to talk about (the problem you addressed or the general topic). Then list the individual points in the order you will present them. Now you may present your information. Keep to the order you announced, and do not stray away from the main message. The body of the presentation will probably take up one half to two thirds of the time at your disposal.

Before closing, it helps the audience if you briefly repeat the main points again. Do not add any new information at this stage. Show the audience that you have reached the end of your speech by stating your objective once again, perhaps in question form (e.g. Now, do you agree with me that ...?). Alternatively you might encourage a discussion by speculating about what should be done next. End by thanking the audience and inviting questions, when appropriate.

Visuals The purpose of visuals is to facilitate communication. Unfortunately, too many speakers use them to the opposite effect. How often are we treated to innumerable, overcrowded, illegible slides, read word-for-word in a dreary monotone by a speaker whose back is turned to us, while we battle in the darkness against impending sleep? Avoid the temptation to write everything on slides instead of using paper or cards as a reminder of what you want to say.

Before making a visual, always ask yourself if it will simplify and support communication with the audience. Keep the opening and closing phases of the presentation free from visuals. Those you use in the body of the speech should preferably be graphics or life photos rather than text or tables; they should be legible from the back row of the auditorium; and each should contain only a single message. If a visual tends to become overcrowded, split the information into smaller portions. In this way you can reduce the risk of misunderstandings and of being distracted from your audience as you try to manipulate the pointer.

The main types of visual used in scientific presentations are slides and overhead projector transparencies; computer displays are also becoming popular. The overhead projector is a modern version of the blackboard and should only be used in a small auditorium. Its main advantages are that it does not require a darkened room nor a projectionist, and transparencies can be made simply, quickly and at low cost. Slides, if made and used correctly, leave a more professional impression and are easier to transport. Responsibility for the quality of projection, however, is also shared by the projector, the projectionist, the screen and room lighting as well as slide design.

Visuals for projection should be designed especially for

that purpose. Illustrations from print media are highly unsuitable. The rules for designing slides and overhead transparencies are the same:

- Make all slides in a landscape (horizontal) format. In this way they can be projected to fill the screen. If you use the portrait (vertical) format at the same magnification, the image will extend above and below the screen, or at least the bottom of the picture will be out of the view of people in the back rows!
- Lay out the information to fill the available space, except for the outer 20%. In other words, if you use DIN A4 paper to lay out a slide, the sides of which are in a ratio of 2:3, prepare all artwork within an area 16x24 cm. This allows the photographer to use a standard camera setting to produce slides with a uniform appearance and to avoid hiding information under the slide frame. Photograph people and objects close up, keeping the part you wish to show close to the centre, and avoiding a distracting background.
- Label clearly with large, simple sans serif lettering (e.g. Helvetica, Univers or similar typeface). Write horizontally and use capital letters sparingly (for proper names and at the beginning of sentences). Do not split words, do not underline and do not use abbreviations that might lead to confusion. Lettering is large enough if you can read it directly from the slide without magnification!
- Choose colour combinations and patterns carefully to ensure maximum contrast.
- Present information accurately. Check spelling and numbers; do not manipulate scales to exaggerate differences.

The abstract The abstract for an oral presentation may be longer than what is usual for publications and may also contain tables and figures. Otherwise, the same rules apply. Conference organisers often supply special forms on which you should prepare the abstract in camera-ready form.

Handouts Since your presentation is not as detailed as a written paper, you may want to provide a handout for interested listeners. This may consist of an extended version of your abstract plus additional tables and copies of your slides.

Remember to put in the names and addresses of the author(s), and the name, date and place of the meeting where the paper was presented. You could also put this handout on Internet. Don't forget your own e-mail address, so that interaction is made as easy as possible.

Delivery

The way you deliver the information is just as important as what you say. It is therefore essential to take every opportunity to practise before the day. Make sure you can deliver the presentation in the allotted time, preferably less. Videotaping rehearsals is an excellent way to get an objective feedback on the overall effect.

Before your session starts, make yourself familiar with the equipment and the acoustics. Are your slides in the right order and the right way round in the projector? Do you have to operate the projector and the light switches yourself or is there a projectionist? If you use a microphone, how sensitive is it? Is it fixed, or does it move with you? With a fixed microphone you will have to be particularly careful about being understood when you turn your head, for example, to look at slides.

Though your pulse may be racing, your hands sweating and your legs shaking, show that you are in command of the situation. Speak standing up and to the audience (not over their heads, to the lectern or to the screen). Look at the people in the audience and show enthusiasm for your subject; smile and be assertive, but be careful about telling jokes. Humour can easily become offensive or distract from your topic. Speak slowly, articulating the words clearly and loud enough for everyone to hear. Keep sentences short and simple, and use the active voice. Avoid jargon.

Display each visual long enough for its content to be understood, or as long as you talk about it, whichever is longer. But remove the slide before you move on to the next topic. If the next topic has no visual, insert a blank slide to bridge the gap until you need the next visual. Do not show slides that distract from what you are saying, and do not put on the lights between slides. If you need to use a pointer, hold the light steady. Waving it around may hide your shaking hand, but serves no useful purpose. By using simple visuals, a pointer becomes unnecessary. See Box 12.2 for a summary.

Box 12.2 Checklist: Preparing an oral presentation

Aim	√
Audience	√
Main points	√
Body	√
Opening	√
Close	√
Visuals	√
Abstract	√
Handout	√
Rehearsals	√

Poster presentations

To communicate effectively on a poster, you need to combine certain aspects of preparing a written paper with some of those required for oral communication. Most visitors to poster sessions walk slowly round the room, glancing quickly at each poster to see if it might interest them. The first duty of a good poster is therefore to attract attention and to communicate its main message in a few words. As most people pass by at a distance of more than one meter, lettering must be large enough to be legible at such distances.

Like an oral presentation, a poster can only show the main highlights of a study, but the structure is more like that of a written paper. Show data graphically, if possible. Illustrations may be in portrait format if that fits better into your layout; they should be kept simple and labelled horizontally as for slides, but be independently understandable with title and legend, as for publication. Putting references into the text in the Harvard style has the advantage that readers, who are probably familiar with your subject, will recognise the reference. Then you can save space on the poster by listing details of the references only on the handout. The abstract and the handout for a poster are similar to those required for oral presentations.

Preparation Obtain details as early as possible about the allowed length and breadth of the poster, possible methods of fixing, any formal restrictions regarding layout and design, etc. Prepare an outline of the content, using a clear structure. The title should be short and meaningful. Instead of the usual headings (introduction, methods, results, etc.) introduce each section with a short informative statement like those used by journalists. Select and design the illustrations and then write the text, keeping it as brief and simple as possible.

Next draw a plan of the layout approximately to scale to see if everything will fit in without making the poster overcrowded. Plan to write the title in a type whose capital letters are at least 30 mm tall, so it is legible from 3 to 4 meters distance. Subheading capitals should be at least 10 mm tall, those in the text at least 5 mm. Make sure that readers can find their way through the text without difficulty. Put the illustrations close to where you refer to them in the text and number them. If you plan to fit the poster on to several cards, calculate the appropriate size and number of cards required. For ease of mounting in the hectic of the meeting, number them in the correct order. If the poster will be printed on one sheet, lay out the information in columns with the text justified to the left and without splitting words. Leave adequate margins round the edge and between columns. If posters are to be numbered, put the number as it will appear in the programme above the title.

Production and display The most convenient way to produce the final version is on a computer using appropriate layout and graphics programmes. Photographs can be scanned in or attached after printing. The whole poster can be printed as one A0 sheet using a professional large format colour printer. These can often be found in graphical service organisations and this will produce a professional looking result at relatively low cost. If you don't have a computer at your disposal nor the funds to have the poster produced professionally, choose between rub-down or adhesive lettering, stencils or careful handwriting. Failing all else, you might use a typewriter with an 18-point type for the normal text.

Choose an open typeface that is easy to read. That

might be a roman typeface such as New Century Schoolbook or a sans-serif typeface like Helvetica. Avoid ornate and cursive typefaces. If you need variation, you may combine a roman type (e.g. for the text) and a sans-serif type (for headlines), but you should never combine different typefaces of the same class. Distinguish legends from the main text by using a larger or smaller size of the same type. Avoid writing whole words or sentences in capital letters; it reduces legibility. Underlining has the same effect. Colour can increase the attractiveness of your poster if used carefully. It can also have the opposite effect if misused.

It is a good idea to make two copies of the poster if possible, in case one gets damaged or lost. Also make sufficient copies of the handout. It should be designed and produced with the same care as the poster. There are many ways to fix posters to the display wall; test the method you plan to use beforehand. Take plenty of fixing materials with you to the meeting, including scissors and alternative materials such as pins and adhesive tape. You never know whether you will find different conditions from those you expected when you arrive. Finally, be at your poster during the poster session to answer questions and to distribute handouts.

13

The Clinical Study Report

Nicola La Grue

Introduction

The primary aim of any clinical trial is to allow the investigator and/or pharmaceutical company to collect data to answer one or more questions concerning the investigational products. Often the most urgent priority at the end of the trial is to process the data and analyse it statistically, in order to use the results to make decisions about further research. For trials that are not part of a confidential drug development process leading to market, speedy and open communication to other research workers and institutions is achieved through oral and poster presentations and journal publication (see chapter 12). However, for trials which will comprise part of a dossier for submission to a regulatory authority, a thorough, well written and accurate report of the entire study and its results is vital. In fact, it is considered good practice to prepare an integrated clinical study report (CSR) for all clinical trials, including those terminated early for whatever reason.

What is a CSR?

The report is a single document that gives a complete picture of the clinical trial from beginning to end, much as any student would produce for an experiment in a laboratory. It explains the methodology and actual conduct of the trial, it provides a description of the data management and statistical analysis, it discusses the results and conclusions, and most importantly it addresses the objectives of the study. The report may be as little as 50 pages long, for example in the case of a 6-patient pilot study. Or it may be thousands of pages long - normally the case for large studies with hundreds of patients which generate huge data listings.

The need for accuracy and clarity in a CSR cannot be overemphasised. Obviously, if the analyses are incorrect or unsuitable, or the results interpreted wrongly, future research may be shaped in an inappropriate direction. However, failure to present results clearly can be equally costly - promising results may be hidden or a critical costly - promising results may be hidden or a critical adverse effect may go unnoticed. Because of the importance of the CSR, rigorous quality control measures should be used in its preparation. Many companies also insist on a quality assurance audit of the clinical study report.

Who writes the CSR?

The Company or the Investigator himself may be responsible for writing the report. The Investigator will certainly want to review, if not write, the clinical section.

The CSR may be an integrated document comprised of sections written by several different specialists, e.g. pharmacokineticists, statisticians etc. However, this may lead to inconsistency and repetition and make the final report difficult to read. The best solution is for one person to act as the main author and to seek input and review by the relevant experts. The author may be the investigator but many pharmaceutical companies now employ specialist Medical Writers. Medical writing is an unusual, relatively new profession, requiring the peculiar mix of an enquiring scientific and logical mind, and excellent written skills with attention to detail. The writer must be able to understand all that goes into the report in order to present and summarise it well; to this end a sound understanding of basic statistics and pharmacokinetics is necessary, as well as a fair amount of clinical knowledge.

Report format

There is an International Committee on Harmonisation (ICH) guideline for the preparation of CSRs, the general content of which most companies now follow. Certain sections may be tailored depending on the nature of the trial and investigational products, but the generalised standard sections are presented in Box 13.1. The guideline also suggests that copies of critical study-related documents are incorporated as appendices to the CSR, in addition to the data listings for the subjects who took part in the trial; a list of these documents is provided in Box 13.2.

A brief synopsis must also be prepared for each report; this is actually part of the report and should contain key details of the study methodology, together with the results and conclusions reached in the main body of the text. The synopsis is usually about 3 pages long and contains numerical data and not just text or p-values. The ICH guideline also gives us a standard format for the synopsis (Box 13.3).

How to approach writing a CSR

Nowadays authors have to be computer literate. The report text, tables and figures are all usually handled electronically, and report templates often demand expert skills in word processing packages. Once the computing side has been addressed, the author must become completely familiar with the available study documentation; usually the protocol and case report form will be used as the starting point for the report methodology sections. A good author will be able to picture the study procedures, so that he/she can communicate them clearly in a report. Protocols may be ambiguous in certain places and writers should be encouraged to speak with study personnel to determine exactly what procedures were followed. In addition, it is important to note that when describing the study methodology it is not enough simply to regurgitate the study protocol (see chapter 6). The author must document, as far as possible, what actually happened; if it differed to what was planned this should be stated and any consequences discussed.

The Results sections are usually compiled after the Materials and Methods sections have been drafted. Close liaison with the statistician, pharmacokineticist and medical adviser is required to ensure the results are presented and summarised accurately. Again, if the actual analyses differed to those that were planned at the study design stage, this must be explained. Data management and statistical analysis is examined more closely in chapter 7 and 8.

Finally, the Discussion and Overall Conclusions need to be drafted. The efficacy and safety results should be briefly summarised and discussed but care must be taken not to simply repeat previous sections, nor to introduce new results. New and unexpected findings need to be clearly identified and comment should be made on their significance. The results also need to be discussed in the light of other existing data. Any specific benefits or special precautions required for individual subjects or at-risk groups should be highlighted. Implications of the results for future studies should be identified.

Ultimately, the conclusions of the report must address the study objectives defined in the protocol. If the study has been well designed, the report will provide a vital stepping stone to the future development or marketing of the investigational product.

Review and finalisation

Ideally, once the report is in a complete draft form, it should be reviewed by several key personnel including all the contributors and the Principal Investigator. The author will liaise with the reviewers as necessary, ensuring sufficient discussion and agreement on key conclusions, before collating the comments and updating the report accordingly. Depending on the extent of changes, further drafts may be necessary, but ultimately a final report should be produced in as timely a manner as possible, certainly no more than 6 months after the end of a trial. The final report must be signed by at least the Principal Investigator or Sponsor's responsible medical officer (see Box 9.4 for an example signature page), and copies sent to any other main investigators at other study centres which participated in the trial. A copy of the report or synopsis should also be sent to the Ethics Committee(s) which approved the study protocol.

Box 13.1 Table of contents proposed by ICH guideline

1. TITLE PAGE
2. SYNOPSIS
3. TABLE OF CONTENTS FOR THE INDIVIDUAL CLINICAL STUDY REPORT
4. LIST OF ABBREVIATIONS AND DEFINITION OF TERMS
5. ETHICS
   - 5.1 Independent Ethics Committee (IEC) or Institutional Review Board (IRB)
   - 5.2 Ethical Conduct of the Study
   - 5.3 Patient Information and Consent
6. INVESTIGATORS AND STUDY ADMINISTRATIVE STRUCTURE
7. INTRODUCTION
8. STUDY OBJECTIVES
9. INVESTIGATIONAL PLAN
   - 9.1 Overall Study Design and Plan Description
   - 9.2 Discussion of Study Design, including Choice of Control Groups
   - 9.3 Selection of Study Population
     Including inclusion/exclusion criteria and removal of patients from therapy
   - 9.4 Treatments
     Including details of the investigational product(s), method of assigning patients to treatment groups, selection and timing of doses, blinding, prior and concomitant therapy and treatment compliance
   - 9.5 Efficacy and Safety Variables
     Including details of the efficacy and safety measurements, including the primary efficacy variable(s), appropriateness of measurements and drug concentration measurements
   - 9.6 Data Quality Assurance
   - 9.7 Statistical Methods Planned in the Protocol and Determination of Sample Size
   - 9.8 Changes in the Conduct of the Study or Planned Analyses
10. STUDY PATIENTS
    - 10.1 Disposition of Patients
    - 10.2 Protocol Deviations
11. EFFICACY EVALUATION
    - 11.1 Data Sets Analysed
    - 11.2 Demographic and Other Baseline Characteristics
    - 11.3 Measurements of Treatment Compliance
    - 11.4 Efficacy Results and Tabulations of Individual Patient Data
      Including results of the analysis of efficacy, statistical/analytical issues, drug dose and drug concentration relationships to response, drug-drug and drug-disease interactions, efficacy conclusions
12. SAFETY EVALUATION
    - 12.1 Extent of Exposure
    - 12.2 Adverse Events

Box 13.2 Appendices proposed by ICH guideline

Study Information

- Protocol and protocol amendments
- Sample case report form
- List of IECs or IRBs (plus the name of the committee Chair is required by the regulatory authority)
- Representative written information for patient and sample consent forms
- List and description of investigators and other important participants in the study, including brief curricula vitae or equivalent summaries of training and experience relevant to the performance of the clinical study
- Signatures of principal or co-ordinating investigator(s) or sponsor's responsible medical officer, depending on the regulatory authority's requirement
- Listing of patients receiving test drug(s)/investigational product(s) from specific batches, where more than one batch was used
- Randomisation scheme and codes (patient identification and treatment assigned)
- Audit certificates (if available)
- Documentation of statistical methods
- Documentation of inter-laboratory standardisation methods and quality assurance procedures if used
- Publications based on the study
- Important publications referenced in the report

Patient Data Listings

- Discontinued patients
- Protocol deviations
- Patients excluded from the efficacy analysis
- Demographic data
- Compliance and/or drug concentration data (if available)
- Individual efficacy response data
- Adverse event listings (by patient)
- Listing of individual laboratory measurements by patient, when required by regulatory authorities

Case Report Forms (CRFs)

- CRFs of deaths, other serious adverse events and withdrawals due to adverse events
- Other CRFs submitted (as considered appropriate)

Box 13.3 Report synopsis format

<table>
<tr><td>Name of Sponsor/Company:</td><td colspan="2">Individual Study Table Referring to Part of the Dossier</td><td>(For National Authority Use only)</td></tr>
<tr><td>Investigational product(s):</td><td colspan="2">Volume:</td><td></td></tr>
<tr><td>Active ingredient:</td><td colspan="2">Page:</td><td></td></tr>
<tr><td colspan="4">Title:</td></tr>
<tr><td colspan="4">Principal Investigator/Investigators</td></tr>
<tr><td colspan="4">Affiliation (if different to study centre):</td></tr>
<tr><td colspan="4">Study centre(s):</td></tr>
<tr><td colspan="4">Analytical site (if applicable):</td></tr>
<tr><td>Studied period:</td><td colspan="2">Date of first enrolment:
Date of last completion:</td><td>Phase of development:</td></tr>
<tr><td colspan="4">Objective(s):</td></tr>
<tr><td colspan="4">Methodology:</td></tr>
<tr><td>Number of subjects:</td><td>Planned:</td><td colspan="2">Analysed:</td></tr>
<tr><td colspan="4">Diagnosis and main criteria for inclusion:</td></tr>
<tr><td colspan="4">Test product: [dose and mode of administration, batch number]</td></tr>
<tr><td colspan="4">Reference product(s): [dose and mode of administration, batch number]</td></tr>
<tr><td colspan="4">Duration of study drug treatment:</td></tr>
<tr><td colspan="4">Criteria for Evaluation:

Pharmacokinetics/Pharmacodynamics:
Efficacy:
Safety:</td></tr>
<tr><td colspan="4">Statistical methods:</td></tr>
<tr><td colspan="4">Pharmacokinetic evaluation/Pharmacodynamic results:
Efficacy results:
Safety results:

Conclusion:</td></tr>
<tr><td colspan="4">Date of report:</td></tr>
</table>

Box 13.4 Example signature page

Principal Investigator's Signature
Title:
Authors:
I have read this report and confirm that to the best of my knowledge it is a true and accurate account of the conduct and results of this study as performed by [ ] in compliance with the Guideline for Good Clinical Practice, ICH Harmonised Tripartite Guideline.
Principal Investigator: Date:

14

Clinical research in a developing country

Alfred van Meurs and William Howlett

Introduction

The principles of clinical research in a developing country are not different from those in a developed country. Every study must have clear objectives, a satisfactory study design and analysis and be ethical. The essential steps necessary for conduct of successful research described in detail in other chapters of this book are similar in this situation. For example, a protocol should answer to the same standards wherever the research is taking place. These aspects will therefore not be further discussed here again.This chapter will not be a repetition of other chapters of this book set in a sunny climate!

There are many difficulties in carrying out clinical research in developing countries by comparison with developed countries. Not least are those arising from the obvious discrepancy in resources and manpower. The burden of extra workload, the logistics of transport, the inadequate laboratory facilities, the difficulties of communication are all too familiar to the researcher in developing countries. Even when adequate resources are available, the implementation of clinical research very often requires special practical and adaptive skills peculiar to that developing country. The reward from research in these circumstances stem from the importance of the issues. Typical health problems of developing countries are often matters of life and death or serious disability. The gains to be made by the evaluation of interventions, some of which may be relatively simple and cheap, can really 'make a difference'.

This chapter will attempt to discuss some of the ways by which the practical difficulties can be overcome. The chapter is based on the experience of the authors working as a paediatrician and a general physician in a busy clinical setting in Africa. Ethical considerations of research in developing countries are of great importance, so they are dealt with in some detail. Some useful practical information is provided in the second half of the chapter.

From idea to realisation

When first confronted with work in a developing country the clinician, whether indigenous or expatriate, is typically faced with an enormous workload, appalling poverty and a great scarcity of resources. Initially the question of clinical research is not a priority and it is wise at this stage to allow for a period of acclimatisation in order to see where the real problems and the possibilities for research lie.

For example, an initial idea to carry out an investigation of the serious morbidity and mortality of kwashiorkor patients was abandoned when it became clear that the hospital phase of that disease is the terminal stage of a long process with a multifactorial aetiology, primarily based in the community. A serious investigation of such a problem was obviously far beyond our capabilities.

After a period of time and with increasing experience, many questions arise, all of which seem to require immediate answers. Cases may not fit the textbook descriptions of diseases, or inherited therapies may not fit your idea of rational medicine. The potential researcher sees openings and projects in every direction. It is wise at this stage to focus on one set of problems or one line of research. The main research objective must be clearly understood and considered achievable.

Before embarking on a particular line of research it is also wise to consult with colleagues who have long experience of these conditions. In practice, however, not many hospitals in Africa have long term staff or lines of research that extend over years. It may be desirable to establish contact with staff at the local teaching hospital, or the relevant institute of research in that particular developing country or from abroad. The main aim of this is to exchange information and ideas and to avoid any unnecessary duplication. Modern communication by e-mail and internet access (if available through an unreliable telephone network) provide a great help.

Time

Planning, and finding sufficient time for research is essential This particularly applies to expatriate doctors who generally are on 2-4 year contracts. While a longer stay may be necessary for the large or extended field studies, other types of research may well be feasible in the shorter time period. Research in developing countries is notorious for taking much longer than originally planned. This can arise for a variety of reasons, including inadequate planning or unavoidable delays. Some delays are preventable. For example in planning research on a seasonal disorder like kwashiorkor or malaria, a small delay caused by late application or a missed deadline for the ethics committee or the slow processing of a work permit may result in the whole project being delayed by a year.

In addition time is needed for planning and writing, communication with supporting departments overseas (frustrating hours spent on public telephones), travel to research locations, consultations with hospital administrators or other authorities. Time is needed to prepare and deliver lectures about the research to supporting staff. Supervision of data entry, analysis of the data and applying the results are also time consuming. And when all this is going on, one cannot do ward rounds, clinics or operations.

A project is not finished when the last data are collected and analysed. Often, the research will be considered justifiable if its findings can and will be applied to local clinical practice. If inadequate provision is made for this implementation, the local participants will be left with a feeling of betrayal and they are likely to resist any future research proposals.

Some remarks on study design

Epidemiological studies

Epidemiological studies involve the measurement of the distribution and determinants of disease in human populations. They are used to study aetiology, disease distribution, the natural history of disease and for planning and evaluation of a particular intervention. The need for epidemiological studies in developing countries is particularly strong in Africa where observed local disease patterns may not fit the descriptions available in textbooks or medical literature. The most appropriate epidemiological studies in this situation are often *descriptive studies*. These involve describing and measuring the rate of disease by time, place and person in individuals with reference to the population from which they come. These are by far and away the commonest studies carried out in developing countries and are often a prerequisite for any intervention studies to be carried out at a later date.

Analytical studies

Analytical studies are either of the case control or cohort type and involve studying the characteristics of individuals as compared to the populations where the patient normally resides. The *case control* method starts with the identification of a group of cases (with the illness) and controls (without the illness). The prevalence of exposure to a factor is then measured and compared in the two groups. The advantages of this method of study in developing countries are low cost, speed, and ability to study current hypotheses. Also the cases under study may be abundant. Disadvantages include its proneness to selection or observer bias and difficulties in defining and selecting controls.

Cohort studies are generally more complex and involve studying the incidence of disease in a group of persons exposed, and a group unexposed to a potential cause. Advantages are the ability to measure exposure before disease onset and consequently true incidence rates. A major disadvantage in developing countries is expense, particularly if the study is prospective and involves a large population. Costs may be minimised by relying on historical data and using available systems for monitoring disease occurrence such as registries. However disease registries are notoriously inaccurate in many developing countries.

Intervention studies

Intervention studies start with two or more similar groups of subjects, only one of whom has been deliberately assigned to undergo the intervention. All subjects in both groups are then followed in order to assess the outcome of interest. The advantage of this type of study is that it can test a hypothesis and avoid bias and confounding. Such studies pose serious methodological and ethical issues because of the implications of the results of the study for national policy in developing countries. For example, intervention drug trials are rarely performed in developing countries because there are little or no commercial incentives for drug companies to market their drugs there, regardless of outcome or potential benefit.

The study protocol

Objectives

As already outlined in this book careful attention to the study hypotheses and a clear definition of study objectives are among the first steps in any research project. Nowhere is this more necessary than in developing countries where scarce resources demand an even more critical approach. The aspiring researcher is obliged to follow the idea processing steps described in Chapter 1 as carefully as possible. This may lead to the abandonment of many research projects.

Case definition, and diagnostic criteria

Precise diagnostic criteria for the definition of a case are essential. This is particularly the case in clinical disease where inclusion or exclusion criteria may not be so clearly defined. It is wise at this stage to consult the WHO in Geneva where internationally accepted criteria for most diseases are available. Defining the study or reference population is also vital. This again may present particular problems in developing countries where reference populations may not be so easily defined. In the past many tropical diseases have been described from hospital based studies. These reflect highly selected cases, referred to a teaching hospital, and may not reflect the true situation in the non-teaching hospitals and in the community. Clinical (hospital based) studies are easier to conduct but also more difficult to interpret than population based studies.

Ethical considerations

Ethical considerations are of primary importance in developing countries. Obviously they apply more in intervention than in observational studies. It is the responsibility of the investigator(s) to make certain that the study is ethical. The final decisions regarding the ethics of any study are subjective and subject to local circumstances. WHO and the Council for International Organisations of Medical Sciences have published a useful reference on the subject.

A number of general principles apply. Ideally, proposals for research should come from communities themselves and reflect the needs of that community. The priority of a research proposal should be considered within the context of the overall problems facing the community in which it is to be conducted. The community should also have a reasonable expectation of benefitting from the research in both the short term and the longer term. Sometimes the effect of a field trial may be more immediate and obvious or alternatively may be subtle and require careful and balanced consideration before making recommendations. Research projects may also have a number of unsuspected impacts locally, both positive and negative. Positive impacts might be increased jobs, cash flow, and local transport. Negative effects might include increased disruption in local communities and increased disillusionment by the provision of unsustainable health care facilities which deteriorate once the research is completed. A recent example of unethical research in Africa was of HIV surveillance studies being carried out in areas where there were inadequate resources for screening of blood transfusions for HIV. The negative impact of such studies is obvious.

A common form of research in developing countries is the opportunistic or 'hit and run' type of research mainly performed by researchers from rich, developed countries. This type of research has its origin in the knowledge that developing countries are sources of interesting cases and pathology. Under the guise that it is 'for their own benefit' information is collected and later published with no local follow up or intervention in mind. This type of research has obvious negative consequences.

Informed consent

The attitude of doctors towards patients in a developing country can be very directive. This is due to a number of factors, like the enormous case load in clinical practice, the different expectations of modern medicine by the patients, and the differences between doctors educated in the West and illiterate patients with spiritualistic beliefs about health and disease. Information about treatment may be substandard. The danger exists that this attitude persists when conducting research. This should be avoided at all costs, and the principle of voluntary participation after fully informed consent must be adhered to.

All individuals must freely consent to take part in research after being fully informed of the main aims and benefits or hazards of the study. This consent usually takes the form of a signature on a consent form, though in an illiterate population this may take the form of an X. In the case of children or other dependents consent is obtained from a parent or guardian.

In many developing countries there is less emphasis on individual rights and autonomy and this should also be recognised. For example, women will in many instances also need to consult their husband before giving permission to participate.

However, coercion must be avoided and the autonomy of subjects respected. Subjects should be allowed to

Box 14.1

> In one prospective observational study to determine the natural course of anemia in Newborns in Tanzania, the hemoglobin level at which children were taken out of the study and treated was much lower than would be acceptable in a developed country. Despite this, children in the community with this level of anemia would normally go untreated. In this example the seemingly unacceptable practice of observing the natural course of anemia and its attendant morbidity was considered justified by the hope that the study and subsequent analysis will bring improvement in the management of anemia in newborns. Research of this type must be 'operational' and be part of an overall action plan to improve the prevailing conditions.

participate or withdraw from the study without any negative consequences. There should be no undue political pressure to participate. For example it is not uncommon for community based researchers in Africa to be introduced early to the local political and religious leaders. Despite obtaining their support it is still necessary for the researcher to abide by the Helsinki declaration and obtain informed consent from individual participating subjects even though their leaders indicate otherwise.

Confidentiality

It is very important that the confidententiality of the participating subjects be maintained. This may involve restricting the identity and individual results of subjects to members of the research team only. Confidentiality may be a particularly sensitive issue in developing countries because of the worry that information collected could be used against individuals or their community. It may be wise then early on to ensure strict observance to confidential procedures like HIV surveillance.

Incentives

Given the very meagre incomes of most people in developing countries there may be an inclination to reward participants with money or in kind. This is not recommended, although it would certainly increase participation but the reward must be balanced against the inevitable loss of autonomy. Compensation for loss of income due to clinic attendance or for transport may be used as an incentive in certain cases. Non-financial rewards such as free medical treatment are generally seen as more acceptable by the participating group. The provision of treatment for malaria, worms or scabies are successful examples used by the authors.

Determine the best possible treatment The Helsinki Declaration states that patients should always get the best possible treatment. However, the standard 'proven' therapy is often unavailable in developing countries. A further dilemma also arises at this point because the natural course of disease in many developing countries is often determined by other factors, e.g. poverty, poor housing, lack of water, undernutrition, and inadequate medical care (see Box 14.1).

Ethical review committees The proposed research should conform with the standards set by the Ethical Review Committees both of the host country, and of the funding agency, if it is externally funded. Again there is no reason to deviate from Good Clinical Practice.

Where to obtain basic information In order to formulate the research question, it is mandatory to do a full search for existing literature on the subject, and to collect relevant data from local sources. Although this may seem obvious to the researcher with a university library at hand, this is easily omitted or done less thoroughly, when computerised literature service and modern libraries are unavailable. A connection to an academic library is very helpful. Alternatively, an organisation in Liverpool (CHESS: Community Health Support Service. Department of International Community Health. Liverpool School of Tropical Medicine, Pembroke Place, Liverpool L3 5QA, United Kingdom) will do computer searches at a modest price for researchers in developing countries. Internet access has dramatically changed the way information can be obtained, both by being able to reach colleaugues in universities by e-mail and by the availability of useful websites.

The World Health Organisation provides a wealth of information on health and disease of most warm-climate countries (Technical Report series; Bull.of World Health Organisation, World Health Statistics Annual, Weekly Epidemiological Record, and reports of the Regional Offices of WHO). However, a search in international literature about a specific tropical problem in a specific area may yield disappointingly little. This does not mean the information does not exist. Many local reports, investigations, theses etc. never reach international literature for reasons unrelated to their importance. Some suggestions as to where to collect valuable baseline data in a developing country are mentioned here.

- Certain individuals in key political and educational positions may be of great importance to the research.
- Few countries have a reliable ongoing birth and death registration. Population data will usually come from a National Census, carried out at long intervals. These data are often inaccurate, as many groups will have been underrepresented. The tax department is likely to have information on occupation, incomes, size of families, and relative affluence and poverty of certain areas. These data will be found at the site of Central Government.
- Much valuable information about rural or isolated areas in a country may be found locked away, or simply forgotten, in the files or the library of a university. For example, the central laboratory may have records (or they can be construed from reports in file) of diseases, bacterial cultures, drug resistant organisms and malaria surveys.
- In countries with an essential drug programme, or centralised drug purchase and distribution, total monthly or yearly drug use per drug, possibly divided per region, will be available.
- In many countries, hospitals run by non-governmental organisations have had the advantage of continued external funding, and staffing by expatriates, while Government hospitals suffered most from the rigors of the economic decline in the 80's. Record keeping is often one of the first victims, so for reliable records, non governmental hospitals are preferred.
- The missionary doctors and sisters have carried out curative work in an area for decades and have built up a large amount of knowledge about the area and its inhabitants in health and disease. They can provide valuable background information.

Organisation of the study

Local organisation and funding

The research should be embedded in a locally existing organisation. In the case of a clinical trial this would be the hospital, and its governing board. There must be a local colleague who is a full counterpart and if possible even the principal investigator. This serves to help competence building and institutional development, a line of development aid now thought to yield most long term benefits for the host country. The proposal by the joint local and expatriate researchers, should then be submitted to local (hospital) Review Committee, and very often also to a National Research Committee for approval and often also for at least partial funding. Funds for locally initiated and executed research into significant health problems are often available through international agencies. If the request is granted it also signifies the commitment of the host country to the main, external financing organisation.

The order in which the various contacts are made is important. Community or village leaders should not be visited prior to consulting at least the District or Regional Administrator and/or Medical Officer. In many countries there is a political organisation that is organised along similar lines as the civil administration, and this may be even more important. In other cases, it may be necessary to consult with church leaders to obtain cooperation.

In the case of a field trial it is essential to obtain cooperation of people with informal influence, who also may also be better judges of the chances of cooperation within the population. Examples are the village elders, a local priest or imam, a woman's group or a local midwife. Early consultation is essential to judge the reception of a research project and the willingness to cooperate. Obviously, health problems that are of general concern will be received best. Still, some creativity may be needed. For example, a regional medical officer was confronted with obstruction by the - male - village elders when he wanted to do a nutritional survey in an area. Only when he brought down a child with severe kwashiorkor to the beer-hut where the men sat drinking, was he able to elicit some form of cooperation.

The exact study design will depend very much on these preliminary soundings of the community. There should be minimal inconvenience and time claim, because rural people in these countries - and especially the women - can have very busy days. For example, visits to the (research) clinic in town could be made to coincide with market day. Together with a reimbursement for the busfare this would be a nice incentive to cooperate. Home visits must not take place during harvest - indeed, most women will be in the fields from dawn till evening, and often stay there overnight. National and Religious holidays must be taken into account. During Ramadan different meal-times may alter pharmacokinetics. Age and grey hairs are associated with authority in many rural areas. After proper introduction age and gender should no more be a problem, although in many (Muslim) communities female patients can only be examined by female doctors/researchers.

Local staff In any investigation of even modest size local staff must be hired and this may consist of a project coordinator, data entry clerk, a driver and laboratory personnel. Expatriate field staff are best teamed up with local field staff.

Selecting local staff must be done carefully and skilfully. Research projects funded from abroad are often associated with good financial rewards and secondary benefits, so understandably it attracts many people. Many will have excellent papers and references. Good local, possibly independent advice from someone with experience in this area is vital in a world where nepotism is common and paperwork not always what it seems..

It is important to test candidates thoroughly for their professional knowledge and their knowledge of the project-language, to avoid later disappointments. Tribal and (local) language considerations must be taken into account when selecting a field worker.

For the average budget of a research project the post 'local wages', when compared to other items is very small. Nevertheless, wages and recompensation must be somehow be in proportion to the salaries and living standard of the country itself.

There is a strong urge by foreign funded organisations - the large multinational aid organisations are the worst example - to lure skilled people away from their lowly salaried government (or other) jobs with hugely inflated salaries, and naturally, they get a good response. This results in a 'local brain drain', and a collapse of slowly build-up competence in government and local organisations. Local staff must have a contract stating precise duties and rights.

Foreign students can be very valuable in a variety of jobs, often as field worker. The foreign students are usually very motivated, have a strong personal interest (the research period is often a requirement of their university) and by definition an adventurous mind-or they wouldn't be there. There are also dangers: they are usually young and unexperienced, and suffer from culture shock. It is essential that the university in the home country takes the responsibility for some form of preparation.

Training All field workers must get a careful instruction into the aims of the study and the methods used. Lectures may be useful to give some background information, but are inadequate to train staff. They can be much more effectively trained in group sessions by means of role play. The participants take turns being interviewer and interviewed. Questions and answers are commented on by the rest of the group. Because of the transcultural situation this can give rise to many surprises. It should be possible to make alterations to questionnaires as a result of these discussions. The questionnaire should only be finalised after field testing.

Case report forms Some points need to be considered when drafting the questions of a questionnaire or case report form.

- The naming system in a country and other personal data may differ considerably. Children may first carry the mother's family name, and later the fathers. Birth dates and ages may be approximations. For more exact age information, and history taking in rural societies one can draw up a table of events relating to certain years (the year of the drought, the year of the visit of the president). The month can be characterised with events like the rains, the sowing, the harvest, and religious holidays.
- Addresses must be asked in detail. Sometimes people have reasons to conceal their true address. For example, in one study many women who wanted to deliver their babies in the Regional Hospital because of (presumed) better facilities, gave false addresses pretending they lived in town. They could not be found and had to be declared lost to follow up.
- If home visits are intended, precise directions must be asked - but even these can be misleading and it may be best to have a field worker accompany the recruited patient home the first time. For large field studies modern hand-held satellite navigation systems (Global Positioning Systems-GPS), that can now be obtained widely and cheaply, have been used.
- Difference in disease-concept between the investigators and the patients may give rise to

confusion and error, as may the language. For example, in endemic area's the same word is often used for fever and malaria.

Equipment There must be a central office with good accessibility for field workers. Basic office equipment, computers, printers and photocopiers are indispensable tools. Printers and photocopiers need 'mains' voltage. Large voltage fluctuations and power breakdowns are rule rather than exception, so a voltage stabiliser and power back up equipment is needed. Depending on the local situation, it may be better to obtain a generator.

For the same reason, (personal) computers should be of the 'laptop' variety with battery-packs that will provide steady operating power for several hours. They can be charged from the mains when it is functioning, and the charging equipment is relatively resistant to power fluctuations.

Communication There should be very regular contact between field workers and researchers. As telephones may be scarce and often malfunctioning, it is best to have a short regular meeting early in the morning every day. Apart from that, a system to relay messages is needed. The researcher has to participate in the fieldwork and do more or less randomised quality checks of the work very frequently to boost morale and ensure continued good quality of the work in progress. A workday in many tropical countries is a long morning: a very early start, then on until 2 or 2.30 p.m. at the latest. Thereafter, people need time for their own problems and businesses. Do not to try to impose a 'Western' type of work-schedule; it will not work!

Transport Independent transport is very important. There are many possibilities ranging from a four wheel drive vehicle to a bicycle and the optimal mode of transport must be chosen. Good provisions for maintenance must be made. Bicycles and motorcycles could be given or sold cheaply to the local fieldworker at the end of the project as incentives for good job performance (and good maintenance of the bike). Road travel in developing countries can be dangerous.

Laboratory equipment Many laboratory methods are advertised as applicable for field conditions, simply because the apparatus can run on a car battery. However, it is safest to transport the samples and use a fixed established laboratory, rather then use methods that have not been validated. Small portable refrigerators that run on car-batteries or gas tend to break down. A large chunk of ice in a coolbox will keep samples cool a whole hot tropical day long. Samples should be transported in safe, closed containers and subsequently placed in a freezer. In many countries there is good experience with electricity operated and gas operated fridges for vaccine storage because of the successful Extended Programme on Immunisation. Freezers that stay cold are difficult to find. There must be an emergency plan for prolonged power shortage - someone must be 'on call' if it happens in weekends. If samples need to be transported abroad, excellent organisation at both ends of the journey is essential.

The study in progress

If preparation has been sufficient, the work should now proceed satisfactorily. Of course, there are always emergencies. It is important, from the investigators point of view, not to slacken control: keep up the quality control in the field, make sure there are no delays in laboratory work or data entry. Continuous availability and trouble shooting are necessary. The researcher should be a jack of all trades, he is often the only one around who will repair a socket or drive into town for new paper for the photocopier.

Data processing and reporting

Results must be reported back to the field-workers and other participants, and in a suitable manner to the population who made the study possible. This will pave the way to the next step, which is discussing possible consequences of the findings with the authorities, and again with community leaders. Publication of the results in national or international journals must give full credit, by ways of authorship, to the local counterpart.

Further reading

- Hennekens, C. H. and Buring, J. E. (1987). Epidemiology in medicine. Boston: Little, Brown &Co.
- Robinson, D., ed. (1985). Epidemiology and the community control of disease in warm climate countries, 2nd ed. London: Churchill Livingstone.

- Smith, P. G. and Morras, R. H., eds. (1991). Methods for field trials of interventions against tropical diseases: A toolbox. New York: Oxford University Press.
- Tan-Torres Edejer,T. (1999). North-South research partnerships: the ethics of carrying out research in dveeloping countries. British Medical Journal 319;438-441.
- Vaughan, J. P. and Morrow, R. H., eds. (1989). Manual of epidemiology for district health management. Geneva: World Health Organisation.

Index